MORE PRAISE FOR *AFTER COVID*

"Tactical, scientific . . . with an equal dose of wisdom and keen attention to detail. A must-read for anyone living in this unprecedented time . . . a how-to guide to get healthy, cope with the ever-changing world around us, and thrive."

—JODY LEVY, Global Director and CEO
of SUMMIT, Founder of The Milk
Cleanse and NeuroPraxis App

"Inspiring and constructive, details Garcia's long and frightening personal odyssey to overcome the scourge of the coronavirus . . . offers a wealth of intelligence, guidelines, and recommendations for dealing with and recovering from this devastating virus."

—ARNOLD SIEGEL, Founder,
Autonomy and Life

"A fascinating journey by a master storyteller, from life to near-death experience and back again."

—JOSHUA ROSENTHAL, Founder,
Institute for Integrative Nutrition

"Oz Garcia is the first person I turn to when I need the latest cutting-edge information on anything related to nutrition and supplementation. He is always light-years ahead of anyone else when it comes to biohacking your best self."

—KRISTA STRYKER, World-Renowned Fitness
Expert, author of *The 12-Minute Athlete*

"Oz Garcia is the embodiment of grit, humor, and medical genius. His solutions are radical and effective. His stories of thriving through his Covid trauma are breathtaking!"

—BIET SIMKIN, spiritual teacher, author of *Don't Just Sit There!: 44 Insights to Get Your Meditation Practice Off the Cushion and Into the Real World*

"A poignant, heartfelt, and honest approach to healing, and growing, in the face of crisis and tragedy. We all need hope, we all need a point of reference, and we all need resilience to overcome difficult times in our lives, and this book provides them in abundance. Thank you, Oz!"

—JIM POOLE, CEO, NuCalm

"As someone who has done extensive work and research in health and wellness, Oz Garcia is easily the most effective "person"/biohacker/nutritionist I've come across in this space. His combination of knowledge and demeanor is the perfect formula, in my opinion."

—DR. MONA VAND, Leading Pharmacist, Health Coach and Nutritionist

"There are the good wizards and the bad wizards. Oz is the third kind. He simply always goes above and beyond, testing on himself what works and putting modern science and exceptional pragmatism to the service of outstanding health outcomes for a fortunate few. He literally saved my life. I have endless gratitude and affection for his unique talent and true generosity, and really wish for more people to experience his wisdom."

—THOMAS ERMACORA, Urbanist, Technologist and Futurist

"Oz used the extraordinary amount of information about health and biohacking that he accumulated over his professional life to counterattack and defeat the virus that has assaulted our world. Thank you for sharing this information with other long-haul victims of this pandemic."

—STEVE MERINGOFF, Philanthropist, CEO, Meringoff Properties

"A pioneer in the field of nutrition and anti-aging ... this book will bring so much value to the general population. Oz educates in a way that is relatable and practical. He certainly walks the talk."

—BRIAN BLACKBURN, CEO, Xymogen/Wholescripts

"Oz is my go-to health provider, including when my husband contracted severe Covid. Oz talked us through how to treat him from home, keeping him out of the hospital and ensuring that he had the top-of-the-line care nonetheless, using the protocols he developed. The end result was a shorter duration of illness and zero long-term Covid symptoms. It was an absolute lifesaver. We are forever indebted to Oz and so happy he is sharing his knowledge."

—KHALIYA ERMACORA, Cofounder, Falkora, not-for-profit Mental Health and Neurotech Initiative

AFTER COVID

OZ GARCIA

with

HENRY SCHWARTZ

Regan Arts.

First Regan Arts paperback edition, 2022
Library of Congress Control: 2022933762
ISBN 978-1-68245-203-5 (paperback)
ISBN 978-1-68245-202-8 (ebook)
Interior design by Beth Kessler, Neuwirth & Associates, Inc.
Cover by Janine Agro
www.reganarts.com
NY | LA
Printed in the United States of America

To my loving mother, Clara Fuentes Garcia,
who gave me life in so many ways

The funny thing about facing imminent death
is that it really snaps everything else into perspective.

—JAMES PATTERSON

CONTENTS

COAUTHOR'S NOTE

Covid-19 has been one of our biggest challenges in history. It has decimated the lives of untold millions of people, dominated the news, and pushed our health systems to the brink. When Oz Garcia opted to receive a routine surgery in January 2021, before vaccines were available to him, he naively imagined that this potent virus would play no part in his otherwise healthy life.

However, Covid struck, and struck hard, pushing Oz close to death. And when he thought his battle with Covid was finally over, many of the symptoms lingered for months, resulting in a condition that one in three Americans now face: long Covid. Faced with tremendous adversity, Oz had to find a way not only to lift himself out of the depths of his failing health but also to recover from the damage that long-haul Covid wrought.

These are the tools and practices Oz used to recover from long Covid, and also the practices that changed the path he was on. His story is one of renewal, rejuvenation, and reinvention. Covid almost killed him, but the experience gave him the gifts of compassion, gratitude, and a new life of purpose and tranquility. He wrote this book in the hope that the protocols, rituals, and lessons of his recovery and journey will help you with yours.

—Henry Schwartz

INTRODUCTION

I shouldn't be here.

I should have died in the hospital. Or, at the very least, I shouldn't have the strength to share my story. As a survivor of the most lethal Covid-19 virus, Covid pneumonia, and devastating long-haul symptoms, I completed an arduous road back to full health. A large part of my success came from a conscious decision I made to step outside of the conventional medical recommendations. I knew that I did not have time to overcome long Covid with bed rest or the "give it time" method. I devised a plan and it worked. Now, I can share it with confidence so that it may benefit others who have suffered the same fate.

Covid-19 has torn through the world, so much so that even the largest medical institutions have not been able to find effective solutions for every mutation, variant, and symptom—there are simply too many. The virus is still relatively young—even two years on—and any sort of panacea for long Covid side effects, in particular, is nonexistent. However, there are more advanced and alternative treatments available. Medical institutions are just now becoming aware of long Covid's side effects, but right now they are behind in understanding the possibilities of the benefits of alternative treatments that are available. With hospital overcrowding at an all time high, it is understandable that the ultimate goal is survival and discharge—in, out, and *good luck*. Luck only took me so far before I decided that research and preparation were more effective in my long Covid recovery.

Just to remind you of what Covid means in medical terms, I include the CDC's definition: "Covid-19 is a respiratory disease caused by SARS-CoV-2, a coronavirus discovered in 2019." From my experience, Covid, which is how I will refer to it, has tentacles of considerable length, and its reach is clear and devastating.

Consider this: one in three Covid patients suffers from long Covid. This means dealing with health issues also known as "post-Covid conditions," the official name of the illness, which entails feeling any lingering effects for more than a month after being originally diagnosed with Covid. These side effects could eventually pass or persist indefinitely, and there is preliminary research that the virus could attack healthy tissue even after the incubation period of the virus. Thus, the dismissal of patients from the hospital after a Covid diagnosis, without a guide to avoid or mitigate these potential side effects, may be a crippling decision.

In truth, I believe that after I was released from the hospital I knew more than my doctors about how to surmount long Covid, as I began my descent into its depths. At the peak of my illness, their focus was solely on saving my life, for which I am grateful. My focus, and lifelong work, has been all about restoring lives, enhancing lives, and building optimum strength and immunity in the lives of thousands of my clients. At that point, the focal point became myself and the restoration of my own life.

But this is not just about surviving Covid or the Delta variant or the Omicron variant, which has most recently plunged our country into a new period of mayhem. This is about the deadly mutant strains and variants to come and how the body can and must summon up all of its resources to survive. This virus has proven to be highly transmissible, and has only developed more transmission power in each iteration. The first place to look for potential protection is within, through dedicated research and preparation.

In the story that follows, I will be sharing my experience in the hospital, in recovery, and how I survived. This book is about how I rebuilt my immune system and how I healed and strengthened my devastated body. The protocols and plans that I developed for myself, I also believe, will better protect me against the inevitable potential viral hurricanes in the future.

With forty years of a global practice helping patients pursue, maintain, and elevate their own well-being, I woke up one day and had transformed into my own client. I was truly facing death and, in the end, I had to save myself.

I take both a functional and progressive approach to my health practice. My team includes medical staff who have always overseen the entire protocol, including the nutrients and supplements I recommend for my clients.

My programs are always customized for each of my clients, drawing on the most up to date research in nutritional science, diagnostics, genomics, fitness, neuroscience, nutraceuticals, cosmeceuticals, cognitive and immune system enhancement, life extension, and reducing and/or reversing infirmities.

Recently, I was invited to speak at Summit, a symposium in Aspen centered on a variety of disciplines, with some truly remarkable thought leaders. The question I received most frequently was some variation of this: "How do I live longer while maintaining a high or optimal quality of life? How do I resist premature aging and preventable infirmities?"

I have been fielding these questions my entire working life. But now, in the current climate of Covid, these questions have become more complicated. There exists an alphabet soup of novel viral infections, and the general public is vastly unprepared for them. The way forward comes in the form of crucial adaptation and change in most of our lives, shifts in practice, and wellness expansion. That is what this book is all about.

1

I Went in for Surgery
and Left With a Killer Virus

Until my battle with Covid began, I was in amazing shape. I kept up with a global client base, spoke at bio-hacking events and engagements, and kept up my own high-intensity fitness regime. But, when this virus completely shut me down, I realized my immune system was not programmed for this sort of attack. I realized that living longer, with a high quality of life, would require an exceptional amount of rebooting. Fortunately, having previously taken care of myself and my body, it gave me a leg up and I was able to understand how to rebuild myself and to then offer my insight to help my clients face equally formidable challenges.

Everything I have ever taught my clients has been based on decades of study, practice, and research. Of course, physical fitness and exercise have always been included in any plan. But in maintaining my own fitness regime—forty years of running, racing, and marathons—I have accumulated my fair share of sports injuries. I had kicked the can down the road long enough and I knew it was time for me to correct some of my injuries as they had begun to be unsustainably painful.

So, I scheduled the first of what was supposed to be a number of surgeries for the first week of January 2021. As it turned out, the Covid vaccine was about two weeks from being widely available to my demographic.

In retrospect, I really should have postponed the surgery until the vaccine was available, just to be as safe as possible. However, at that time in my life, I denied the reality that "it"—contracting Covid and ultimately suffering from it—could happen to me. I now look back at my previous self and realize how foolish I was to think that I would be "safe" in the hospital at a time of mass infection in the largest city in America.

Working with a unique team of neurological surgeons at New York City's Mount Sinai Hospital, I went full speed ahead into a surgery, one that I knew was necessary, smack dab in the middle of a Covid surge and a brand-new, dangerous variant. The surgeons had decided to divide up the surgeries into four quadrants that would take place over several months, beginning with my neck and working down my body.

After the initial surgery, I shared a recovery room with a young international rugby player, who I later learned was living it up while I slept. This fellow had traveled from abroad for surgery, and every time I'd wake up, there were other guests floating in and out—all unmasked. In my daze, I remember this pleasant fellow coming over periodically to chat with me. In retrospect, I concluded he, or one of his guests, had to have been my patient zero who brought Covid, the Delta strain, into my life.

After a brief and hazy two days in the hospital, I asked my doctor to discharge me. I was concerned because adequate safety precautions were not in place, and I began to worry about the growing viability that I may become infected. Once I got home, I felt deeply lethargic with incessant systemic pains all over my body. After five days of this intense aching, and my neck killing me, I thought perhaps something had gone wrong with the surgery. I called the surgeon's office but they did not have much for me. "Wait it out," they told me. "You're just in recovery."

Instead of relying on pharmaceuticals or painkillers, which I do not take, I took ice baths and used hot compresses, but found no relief with either. After masking up, I made it to my office later that week, but, after practically keeling over, someone drove me home around 5:00 p.m. I do not remember anything until I woke up, in the same clothes I had worn to the office, at 4:00 a.m. on Sunday morning. I had slept through the entire weekend. The only thing I remember thinking was, *This is one hell of an awful recovery*. By Tuesday, with still no relief, I called the neck surgeon and told him that it was an emergency and I had to see him right away.

While complimenting his own workmanship on my neck, the surgeon quietly remarked, "*You wouldn't mind going over to the Covid ward.*"

Not a question, simply a statement.

The surgeon's team ran a PET scan and found two clots in my right leg, and as I quickly learned, the clots were a product of Covid and potentially lethal. To that point, I had not thought about Covid because I did not have any of the documented symptoms, aside from deep exhaustion, which I attributed to recovering from surgery. Even though I had felt incredibly ill in the days following surgery, I could not have fathomed that it was anything other than "general recovery pain."

Shortly afterwards, I found myself surrounded by doctors in a room with tall glass windows. I watched people coming in on gurneys and remember thinking, *This is not good.* It was not the type of hospital room that I ever expected to occupy. The preliminary tests revealed that I was not only positive for Covid, but also that my lungs were filled with micro clots indicating Covid pneumonia. My oxygen levels plummeted down to 68 percent. Sensing the conditions of the hospital quarters, I quickly suggested to the team that I go home and quarantine. I was met with immediate disbelief, and so began my almost three-week detention in the hospital.

THREE WEEKS IN COVID HELL

For any Covid skeptics out there, let me tell you the details of what I refer to as my personal hell. It began with what my doctor had meant by the "Covid ward." Due to the patient overload at the hospital, I would be receiving treatment in a converted medical storage room, one that I would share with several anguished patients, often screaming for help. The gravity of my foolish choice to receive elective surgery at that time weighed heavily upon me. While the reality of my situation began to reach an uncomfortable apex, this was only a fragment of my growing awareness of what this virus might do to my body and mind.

In the time I was hospitalized, two of my fellow room-mates in the storage room died in beds on both sides of me. With Covid hospitalizations at another sudden high, the best I could get, with the help of my outside concierge doctor, was a move to a more "elite" storage room.

Even in a more desirable storage room, white light blared throughout the room at all hours of the day, making any rest nearly impossible. Even in the rare instances I could find sleep, nurses would wake me up three or four times a night to draw blood, take my blood pressure, check my oxygen levels, and make sure I was still alive. It was now early February, and I had been in a hospital storage room for almost three whole weeks.

I had always been a strong, lean man with no body fat, but my work ethic and lifetime of dietary discipline and exercise proved to be insufficient in the fight against Covid. I lost thirty pounds in sixteen days and could count my bones. I had rapidly disintegrated into a skeleton with hanging skin.

At a certain point, the pulmonary team of five doctors wanted me on a mechanical respirator. I refused but, unbeknownst to me, they called my brother and my business partner to get permission. I knew the statistics—only two out of ten Covid patients who require a respirator come out alive. Even if I were to survive, my quality of life could still be miserable. The process of sedating me, inserting a tube into my lungs, and keeping it there for an indefinite period was simply out of the question. I knew the extreme damage that could occur to the brain and respiratory system and I was willing to take my chances with the next best option, and possibly live or die by that decision, as long as it was my decision.

Instead of a respirator, the medical staff attached me to a high oxygen flow ventilator, a breathing device, and an oxygen tank that provided 100 percent oxygen at sixty-five liters per minute. Picture sixty-five milk bottles filled with oxygen. It was intimidating, but I was clearheaded enough to know that it would beat out any of the severe side effects that could follow the use of a mechanical ventilator. I was also administered the antiviral remdesivir and dexamethasone, a steroid used to bring down inflammation in your lungs.

My prior health routines that I had religiously adhered to in my daily life had completely shut down.

My life, as I knew it, was over. My entire world was now my hospital bed. I was constantly assaulted by the combination of the incessant lights and the humming of the machines that monitored me and kept me alive. It made the healing power of sleep nearly impossible. The television was almost always on in the room. I felt as though I had viewed every episode of *Shark Tank,* in addition to every show on CNN, CNBC, and Fox News. It was a constant barrage of needless, meaningless information and it served as a poor distraction from what I was enduring and attempting to survive.

In moments of lucidity, I knew, even from my hospital bed, that if I were to beat this part of Covid, I would undoubtedly still have a battle ahead of me to regain my former self, by myself. To that end, I began, in my daze, searching for any and every approach and treatment available online. I looked for anything that might possibly help me once I could get home. I also tried to listen to audiobooks, podcasts, anything that could prepare me for the next steps. I told myself over and over that I would make it out of the hospital alive. I just could not predict what condition I would be in. I certainly never suspected that I would be a long hauler.

As I think back now, this calamitous experience triggered an unexpected turning point in my life. My value system had been flipped on its head. I had no idea on what or whom I could rely, what had happened, and what even mattered as I entered a fevered state of mind.

While in the hospital, one of the most precious and meaningful moments occured when one of my dearest friends visited and brought me Jell-O. This small act of kindness immediately brought me to tears. It brought into sharp contrast the fact that, while my energy was focused on trying to stay alive, my mind and thoughts would drift to getting back to the life I had, even as it was unraveling. My thoughts went from trying to survive to thinking about returning to work. I was so conditioned to work, and honestly I was so fucked up, that I was trying to save my company while I was teetering on the brink of death.

I was still trying to hold up the facade that I was okay. It was absurd, but I was still trying to protect my ego. I was losing my life but I was focusing on my vainglorious pursuits. What I really needed, at that time, was peace of mind. For me, that wouldn't come for a long time.

As I became increasingly desperate, I knew I needed a plan to accelerate being discharged. I was determined to get out as soon as I could. The quickest way for me to go home would be by sufficiently rebuilding my lung capacity, which had been the primary reason I had stayed for so long. To that end, I knew I had to get my hands on certain products. Most notably, it would be supplements I had researched that I knew would improve my condition.

On my birthday, I had friends wrap my supplements up as gifts, so that they wouldn't raise suspicion, and had them dropped off at the hospital. Having been told I would likely be hospitalized for anywhere from six to eight weeks, I'd already started my recovery plan from my hospital bed. I had tried time and again to procure supplements from my doctors that I knew would help my recovery—but they were focused on saving lives in an extreme emergency setting, not on restoring the health of those lives.

I told them that in my experience certain supplements could help.

Vitamin D?

No evidence, they said.

Vitamin C?

No evidence.

How about N-Acetyl-Cysteine, also known as NAC, a supplement used to loosen thick mucus and improve lung function and even help repair the brain from injury?

No evidence.

I believed strongly that they were wrong. NAC came to prominence in the 1980s as a supplement within the gay community and was used for individuals who were HIV positive and had developed full-blown AIDS, perhaps along with PCP pneumonia. I knew that NAC would improve my condition. I had spent my life's work studying these supplements.

Every suggestion I raised was rejected by the pulmonologist who slammed his hand on my oxygen device and said, "Only two things are going to get you out of here—this machine and time."

And he walked out.

Without the knowledge of the medical staff, these products, wrapped as birthday gifts, truly helped in my salvation.

I began taking massive amounts of NAC, nitric oxide inducers, zinc, probiotics, and injectable vitamin D. As the days went on, the pulmonologist kept dropping the amount of oxygen, openly admitting how my recovery began to accelerate.

And so it went until he started moving up my discharge date from six weeks to three weeks to a week, and finally, "You could be out of here tomorrow."

It was only on the last day of my hospital stay that a doctor said, "I peeked and saw what you were taking but just be careful with them," to which I responded, "I've got this."

And I got the fuck out of the hospital.

2

My Rough, Rough Road to Recovery

Still catching my breath, and in a dramatically weakened state, I could barely walk out of the hospital and needed the help of a nurse. When I arrived home and slowly passed through my front door, I caught a glimpse of an alien—a ghostlike, wizened old man. For a moment, I was terrified. Was I seeing things? I froze, looked again, and what appeared in front of me was a corpse. The skin on his arms was hanging; the skin on his face was hanging. I didn't know what I was looking at. It was a dead man walking. I had to gather my thoughts because I thought I was hallucinating.

In fact, I wasn't hallucinating. I was looking in my mirror, in my entryway, and the apparition looking back at me, this wizened, emaciated old man, was me.

I stared for a few minutes, slowly comprehending the state I was in, and became completely demoralized.

For a moment, I had no hope, no faith, no belief in a future, and was so overcome with a sense of both terror and exhaustion, it was incomprehensible to me that I could ever feel alive again. I was in the grips of full-blown PTSD and was fully traumatized.

I didn't know what to do and started to cry. I became inconsolable. Just to get into my room was overwhelming. With the help of a nurse, I reached the bed, rolled into a fetal position, and cried for what seemed like hours.

Here I was, the pillar of strength who had spent decades giving others a plan to overcome, a program to deal with their infirmities, the courage to repair their lives, and now I was the one who was completely wasted, physically and emotionally. And it happened in an instant. As a normally energetic person, it was challenging for me to suddenly, in essence, age decades in a few weeks, and become completely dependent on a nurse and a home oxygen tank. Overnight, I had become like a helpless infant.

My first day home from the hospital, I just slept. I slept for the next three days in a row, uninterrupted, except to venture to the bathroom and attempt to eat. I was attached to a home oxygen tank and was dependent on this minimal amount of oxygen at all times for the next month. I went to sleep and woke up to it. The sound of the machine was a constant reminder of my fragile state.

Less than a month prior, my lungs were at peak performance. I was fit enough to do 150 push-ups daily.

Now, I had to be attached to the supplementary oxygen just to get out of bed, sit up, and start whatever activities I needed to perform to stay alive.

I was fortunate to have a nurse-aide, Anna, for my first month out of the hospital. Anna, along with the oxygen tank, were the two morning pillars I could rely on to launch me out of my bed.

My world was the distance I could cover from the bed to the bathroom and, sparingly, I would even make it to the kitchen.

There was only so much energy I had available to accomplish anything that required effort. I'd lost over thirty pounds of muscle, and I felt that lack of strength and power when I tried to do very simple tasks. This produced severe fatigue, sufficient enough to make every single move and gesture painful.

To do anything or to get anywhere, every movement had to be measured.

I spent time in bed calculating the distance to the bathroom and back. Could I make it while walking? Crawling? It usually ended up being some combination of both.

My immediate environment was a landscape fraught with potential peril. If I lost my balance, which occurred often, I'd go flying, and with the loss of padding on my body, I often discovered new bruises.

On one of my first nights home, I suddenly woke up and needed to go to the bathroom. Half asleep and groggy, I went flying headfirst into the floor, momentarily unaware of my own inability to even hold myself up. It must have been three o' clock in the morning. It was pitch black in my room and it took me ten minutes, using all of the little energy I had, to even hoist myself back up onto the bed. I felt that I was at rock bottom, not just in terms of Covid, but of my whole life.

Transitioning from absolute body control to fighting with my own brain to control my limbs was a shift for which I was just not prepared. I went from being a freakish athlete to a rag doll, from moving my limbs at will to having them give up on me. I had been in a partial dream state and had awoken to, frankly, a nightmare. I began to sleep with a night-light in case I fell again or awoke in the middle of the night and forgot my decrepit state. My sleep would continue to be interrupted every night in those early weeks, and incidents like this one continued throughout my recovery.

Even when I began a stricter recovery regimen, I would still suffer from the same anxious outbursts in the middle of the night. I began to eat and sleep well and according to plan—but I would still wake up almost every night in a state of panic. I ultimately realized that this was one symptom of long Covid, coupled with the post-traumatic stress disorder that I had acquired during those three hellish weeks in the hospital.

My panic was completely disconnected from the rest of my waking life. I had been devoting all of my time to developing a path toward some semblance of recovery, but I could not prevent what I eventually came to understand as a frequent amygdala hijack. I had experienced such novel, fearsome moments that my fight or flight response had become disengaged from the rest of my chaotic brain. Covid had caused deregulation within my blood-brain barrier, therefore triggering this dissociative PTSD, from which I still suffer bouts even to this day. These fits still bring me back to my breaking point.

When I would wake up in the morning, I felt as if I had been beaten by a bat. I had such aching, painful muscles and joints, and just turning over to get out of bed was a trial. Remember, in addition to the Covid that hit me, I was also recovering from neck surgery so it was a double whammy.

Even with the painful effects of my various injuries, I had been working out in some capacity just before I had the surgery. Running has always been my number one elixir. Since my early twenties, it had been the cure-all that healed my near-constant anxiety. A lifelong obsessive runner, it had transformed my diet, helped me quit smoking and drinking coffee, and was the main catalyst for me to pursue the career that I still have and love to this day. Covid put an immediate end to any activity, so I lost the chemical boost—the self-generated supply of endorphins, cannabinoids, and euphoria—that had sustained me for decades. Running, too, had also helped me cope with certain childhood traumas, and now the floodgates of unresolved emotion were open and my anxiety returned at an alarming and rapid pace.

In spite of an entire lifetime of training my body to overcome ruminating on past traumas, my internal dialogue, at this point, was uncontrollable, latching onto the slightest thing and keeping me going round and round for hours.

Before the surgery I had ways to fix it, or at least hold it at bay—saunas, ice baths, as much working out as I could possibly do, supplementations—but I needed the surgery to get back to being myself. I needed to rebuild my body. In the process, I ended up destroying it. And I almost lost it for good.

Amidst the supreme desiccation of my body, I felt like a shell of the man I had been—not just because of the loss of physical form but also because of the life I had been leading. Of course, I felt like I had lost the prestige that came with my profession. I have been cited before as a "celebrity nutritionist," whatever that might mean to you. I worked with talented and powerful people. All of them have earned where they are today, and they come to me looking to maintain their body while performing their various occupations at the highest possible levels. Due to this, I lived what is as close to a rock 'n' roll lifestyle as someone my age could. I do not know anyone my age who could have kept up with me—and that is not said lightly, or vainly. I say that because of the hard work I have put into my body and the years of my life I have dedicated to my practice. I had been living within an arrested aging process. For almost fifty years I have been an athlete and trained like one. I started my anti-aging routines after I left college. Luckily, I had the foresight at an early point in my life to look into what it takes to become a healthier human being. But due to the vulnerability of having an elective surgery at the time that I did (before vaccines), I became just as high risk as someone who was immunocompromised or had not put forth even a sliver of the effort I had in anti-aging and maintaining my body. Despite my life's work, I was now in a category of patients that I had never anticipated.

My so-called glamorous, fun-filled, happy-go-lucky life was over. My entire focus was now on survival—learning to breathe, walk, eat, and even wipe my own ass again. I entered the hospital a happy, athletic, vital, and totally autonomous man. I returned a dependent, sick, weak, anxious, fearful, and, as one nurse called me, "elderly" man.

I never saw myself as those things because I have lived, as an adult, an extremely healthy, positive life. For whatever reason, perhaps through my own vanity and delusion, I never considered the possibility of a sudden illness, or having a near-death experience.

My new reality, I must admit, gave me a new level of compassion for the suffering of others. I am ashamed to admit that my own ignorance and blindness did not allow me to *truly* understand what the aging process did to others, even to my own mother, whom I loved dearly. My mother passed away in January 2020, just missing the pandemic. Her passing started my deep grieving and regret for what I perceived to be my lack of understanding as her body aged and broke. It took time and contracting Covid to begin reflecting on what it may have been like for her in her final years.

I deeply regret arguing with her about her own infirmities and degeneration, which included, interestingly enough, chronic pulmonary problems and severe chronic physical pain. I had to go through it myself to understand my mother's suffering. In some ways, I suppose, it was karmic retribution that it ended up happening to me. Were there a time machine, I would do anything to go back and relive that time with her and show her the respect and understanding she needed and required.

Compassion runs on a two-way street. Neuroscience has now demonstrated that compassion is key to both the giver's well-being and to the recipient's. Remember that when taking any journey of healing or spending time with others who have their own challenges. Every day should consist of developing a practice of compassion and forgiveness. Those two are fellow travelers. You must have discipline, grit, patience, ingenuity, fortitude, faith, hope, courage, kindness, a lot of humility, self-control, integrity, perseverance, and trust in yourself. Yes, and trust that you can and will rise above adversity, and come through stronger on the other side of it.

As the days passed at home, I began planning what a day would or should look like. Planning equaled sanity—at least it did in my pre-Covid life. I would look at the day ahead of me and no further. That was enough.

In fact, that was all I was able to do. This was how I began recovering my life. One minute at a time. One movement at a time. One thought at a time. One step, one meal, and then one day at a time.

I knew that I would have to attempt to rediscover a steady routine in my life. I had always found success by maintaining the same habits every day. But now that my body was unrecognizable, and my brain was completely muddled by the virus and my looming PTSD, I needed to look for a solution that wouldn't destroy me. The first step of the solution came from James Clear's inspirational book, *Atomic Habits*.

Clear had suffered a severe high school baseball accident when a player in front of him lost control of his bat, splitting Clear's skull open. Not only was he out of the game but he very well could have been out of life. Despite this massive hardship, with enormous effort and courage, Clear left his college voted as the best and most valuable athlete, and went on to teach people how to build better habits the way he did at the nadir of his recovery process—one small step at a time.

Atomic Habits became my own personal Bible. It taught me how to make small changes, making myself better as little as 1 percent every day. I started by measuring the distance between my bed and the toilet to see how far I could crawl in both directions. I measured every distance, and after months of hard work, I eventually could even do push-ups and sit-ups in my apartment. When I struggled, I would reread Clear's baseline methodology:

Do whatever you can, but have it be a little bit more than the day before.

So, little by little, day by day, I came up with a whole protocol in terms of what I needed to eat, what I needed to do to deal with pain, and, most importantly, how I was going to sleep. I knew the better I slept, the more I would improve, bit by bit. If I wasn't careful with my quality of sleep and what time I went to bed, my whole day was thrown off. My biggest struggle was with energy, and *sleep was my supercharging superpower.* I needed it desperately. I toyed around with countless products, supplements, and devices, the majority of which did not work. But the ones that did, I have included in this book, as they were essential to my recovery.

There were also other parts of my well-being that I had to recalibrate—the main one, besides sleep, was my gut. After just less than a month of subpar hospital food, and the Covid virus in my body, I felt the damage within my stomach. My digestion was absolutely shot and the work I had put into maintaining my bowel and stomach lining had been upended. I knew that the things I would have to eat upon returning home would have to both rebuild muscle mass and my gut microbiome. Food is energy. It powers the body and powers the day. Without adequate sustenance, productivity becomes a fraction of what it could be. Additionally, eating the wrong thing could have sent me spiraling even further. Because of the tenuous state of my stomach, I had to go back to the basics to rebuild—that would be the only way to return to the extravagance and pleasure of what I had eaten before. While my usual eating routine is beyond healthy, it did not provide me, yet, with the nutrients my body so desperately craved. I had to regain cushioning on my body, muscle on my biceps and forearms, anything to make me feel like myself again, to rid me of my new, weakened, skeletal body. I will go into the diet itself later on in the book.

Then there was the state of my mind. I stopped watching the news first thing in the morning. Hearing the news, and all of the negativity it bore, brought me back to my endless, sleepless nights in the hospital storage room. I have been a huge NPR fan (I still am), but I found that even my favorite programs started me out on the wrong foot. I would listen and it would put a sour taste in my mouth and depressing thoughts in my brain. I could feel my anxiety rising with every utterance of Covid and its damaging effects. Even worse, somehow none of it related to my long journey. I supplanted the news media with something that brings me uncapped joy—jazz music. I began to wake up listening to the sounds that had always calmed me, wondering why I had been okay with blaring updates in the morning to begin with. Sometimes I would delve into a podcast that interested me. Anything that would stimulate my brain instead of just filling it with negativity, with rote facts or argumentation. I gave up my subscriptions to the *New York Times*, *Wall Street Journal*, and *Newsweek*. During the day, I might still take some time to read the news, if there was anything important, but it no longer fit into my daily routine, my routine that would push me forward, out of Covid.

I researched endlessly, latching onto any solutions I could in order to keep my spirits up. I began to understand how the depression and anxiety I had been experiencing were also side effects.

I began to schedule daily breath regulation and meditation. My go-to would be a gratitude meditation. Gratitude was the overwhelming sentiment I felt in those first days home. I was grateful to be alive, to the people who helped me, to life, to the knowledge I had, to others who shared their ideas with me, to jazz music, to the healthy food I was able to eat, and acknowledging all that and more was the cure to chronic pain. It was a slight respite in the midst of my journey. Whether I used a meditation device, an aural guided meditation, or some version of my own practice, I would take a short time to live within myself. I would practice five minutes in the morning and five minutes at night, at the very least. Oftentimes, I would go on longer, as it stimulated me in a way that I could not grasp otherwise. I felt fine putting off any other part of my day to turn to a practice of meditation—it was just too important. Gratitude meditation reboots your brain more than anything else I have practiced. I would also write in a gratitude journal. Just ten minutes a day, if that was all I could spare. It became extremely low effort in my life, but its impact was great, and beyond essential for recovery.

I felt hurt by my friends and clients who did not return my calls or texts. Every day I thought I would never get my business or life back. But when I did my meditation, I began to think about what it means to generate a state of loving-kindness to the people I would least care for, working my way up to the people I love the most. It is amazing how it calmed me, and pushed me closer to returning to full health.

In order to offset the effects of my long Covid issues, I never broke this series of rituals and routines. I had spent years studying the brain and different aspects of neurobiology and neurochemistry, so I knew about mindfulness and the absolute necessity of being present and aware of what I was doing. These were very crucial factors for my recovery.

Because I had all the worst symptoms of a long Covid patient, my health was precarious. Two months after my hospitalization, I suffered a pain akin to someone stabbing me in the stomach. I knew the steroids were to blame—they were far too powerful for my damaged body. I had been given dexamethasone, a hugely powerful steroid, one that is often given to horses, mind you, to bring down the inflammation in my lungs. My digestion went to hell. I went from never, ever having a bowel problem to knowing and feeling my bowels were in shreds, completely decimated. Later, a CAT scan revealed a tear on one side of my bowel and the doctors informed me that I needed an antibiotic.

After my search revealed this particular antibiotic's side effects, I then researched my particular kind of tear and I quickly found information that totally contradicted the advice of my doctor. I was fully back to being my own healer. It was pure craziness that this was unknown to the medical professionals. At the time, it felt as if everyone was shooting in the dark, from my original hospital stay to my several visits afterward.

I needed to hit every curative hot button for my digestive system, brain fog, lack of energy, and weight and muscle loss. I needed to modify my eating practices and figure out which probiotics would help heal my gut, bowels, and my anxiety and depression. I am aware that people use marijuana, alcohol, Xanax, Klonopin, and other benzodiazepines to solve their worries—as well as many, many other upsetting "fixes"—but these are temporary forms of distraction and do not fix problems, and might potentially add to them instead.

Despite the abundant overload of information that has and had been taking over the media for months, I cannot inculcate any further my sense of naivete when it came to Covid. Not only do I practice and preach essential skills of anti-aging, and have for decades, but my lifestyle was predicated upon my strong sense of health. I have been an avid runner for forty-five years, never skipping more than two or three days in a row. I had lived like that since the mid-1970s. I had prioritized running over almost everything in my life to this point, so much so that I opted to have surgery in order to get back to running, instead of waiting for the vaccine in the middle of a rampant, killer virus.

My recovery from Covid was exacerbated by my recovery of the surgery that had gotten me into this mess in the first place. I had two major recoveries simultaneously. Moreover, both of them ultimately kept me sedentary for longer than I ever had been. My body function was at an all-time low. All of the kinetic energy I was used to was completely dissipated, and I remained in a constant state of enervation, on top of the general listlessness attached to my specific recovery from Covid.

3

Mature Optimism

The depression and anxiety persisted. I couldn't snap out of it. I was mourning the loss of my old life, and, in retrospect, after working through, baby step by baby step, my recovery from long Covid, I can now admit that I was being self-centered, arrogant, and utterly lacking in a mature, humble response.

The disease took me to my knees, as I'm sure it has many others. I don't want to diminish the seriousness of illness, disease, and the pain and suffering it has caused—but Covid also became my teacher in so many ways. I grew emotionally, intellectually, and spiritually. All that I had valued previously—work hard and achieve, make money, get on the treadmill and acquire, get on the scoreboard, get famous—none of it mattered. *None.*

What begins to happen past a certain point of demoralization and dehumanization is that no matter how much money, fame, acclaim, and ego you have—you come face-to-face with this fact: **a deadly virus does not discriminate**.

When dealing with recovery from Covid, a life-threatening accident, a disease or serious illness, taking personal responsibility for one's own care takes center stage, as it did for me. I learned not to complain, not to whine, and not to feel sorry for myself. I had no choice. I did the research, taking the best from the medical community and the best from progressive, functional medicine and biohacking. I utilized it and paid careful attention to my own care and well-being, and I hope to have the same effect for yours.

Regardless of the challenge at hand, I had to become my own citizen doctor, and I took a highly functional, hands-on approach to my self-care. What is really going to work? As an inquiry:

What could be done to rebuild my lungs?

Could I ever rebuild my body?

How could I protect my brain from the predicted damage?

The more I read and understood the severity of long Covid, the more I refused to buy into the predictions for my condition, what my fate supposedly had in store. I was told, often enough, the litany of what would or could happen to me. Over time, I stopped listening. I would refocus on my own personal cure and lay out my own program regardless of the negative or otherwise distracting noise.

I would try to ignore the bad news and disregard it. I would play over in my head what the doctors told me in the hospital:

Oz, Covid attacked your pancreas and kidneys and, with the severe pancreatitis that you have, you may have long-standing health issues.

I did not wallow in the negativity of these predictions. I did not allow them to define me or my new life.

Oz, with the kind of pneumonia you have, you will likely have permanent scarring that will give you years of difficulty breathing. You will likely not be able to work out again like you once did. You will not be like you were.

I made a conscious decision to think daily that I would take a journey of recovery. I would attain a positive outcome, a full recovery, an affirmative stand, no matter how I felt on any given day.

This was and is one of the key ingredients for making it out of long Covid, and how, incidentally, you make it in life at large. I now refer to this as *mature optimism.*

This virus, and its longer variant, is an agent laying down land mines that may remain dormant and go off at an indefinite, unknown moment. Anyone who has been beaten down with Covid is vulnerable to what can be described as *aftershocks.* Because this is a relatively new virus, as opposed to the common flu or cold, the medical profession has still just begun to understand what patients may experience *post-Covid.* The list to date tops at least one hundred symptoms and counting. It is erratic and often unpredictable.

In fact, we don't yet know if there's going to be a total recovery. Studies are published every day revealing diabetes as a possible side effect, and reports are unveiling potential issues with the pancreas, kidneys, and lungs, to say nothing of the psychological aspects. In an NPR article, Dr. Angela Cheung of the University of Toronto, who is studying long Covid, reported, "If we are conservative and think that only 10% of patients who develop Covid would get long Covid, that's a huge number."

The upshot of my hard work baffled the team of pulmonologists upon a return checkup. Initially, while hospitalized, I had been prescribed Eliquis, a very powerful drug to prevent clots, but one that gave me terrible headaches. When the doctors asked me if I was still on this medication, I replied affirmatively. But the doctor said, "No, no, you've got to stop taking it. You don't have any clots." Actually, I had already weaned myself off the medication and pursued a protocol involving compression devices that I used on my legs, along with a supplemental regimen that I had worked on to stop and dissolve clots. It did wonders for me and I did not have to take Eliquis, which I did not trust.

The checkup also revealed there was only 5 percent scarring on my lungs, and the doctor finished up by saying, "Do whatever you want." He even went so far as to say even people with one lung can run marathons.

I was back at work in three months' time, but it took around six months before I could work efficiently, anything close to approaching my old pace. I began incorporating a category of nutrients called peptides, hyper-progressive nutrients that are novel combinations of amino acids. By figuring out the right peptides to take, I was able to put on all my weight as muscle. I was my own work in progress. The peptides aided the prebiotics, as well as the lung-enhancing devices, breathing tools, and so much more that I will explain later on.

In my line of work, and everyday life, I see too many weakened immune systems, too many health issues, and too many lifestyles that need an overhaul. In the following chapters, I will share my expertise to prepare you for what may come, or what you're going through right now if you have long Covid.

THE VERY BASIC ENTRY POINTS FOR RECOVERY FROM LONG COVID AND HOW TO MAINTAIN YOUR FUTURE PROTECTION

These very basic steps are the ones I took to begin to rebuild my immune system. I had to start somewhere. This part is about vigilance and caution. Even without long Covid, everyone should start here.

- Get vaccinated as soon as possible.
- Wash your hands consistently throughout the day with soap and water.
- Wear the highest quality masks—I recommend the N95, KN95, and KF94.

- Always avoid super spreader events, even those with vaccination requirements.
- Be aware of sleep patterns and follow a schedule with a consistent evening sleep time and a consistent wake-up time.
- Get a physical that includes comprehensive blood work and diagnostic testing.
- Control your diet. Be hypervigilant about what you ingest. Avoid alcohol and too much caffeine.
- Exercise on a regular basis. Even when it feels impossible, do something. Just move your body.
- Do your breathing exercises, with or without devices.
- Get tested often.
- Be mindful.
- Get outdoors.
- Reduce time on your phone, social media, TV, games, and so on, especially prior to bed.
- Journal, either in a gratitude journal or a standard one.
- If possible, work with both a functional medicine practitioner and a general practitioner. Familiarize yourself with their suggestions.

4

My Protocols for Survival

I live and practice in the world of functional well-being, neurohacking, biohacking, and wellness. Functional medicine is often referred to as a form of alternative medicine that focuses on the "root causes" of disease and formulates individual treatment plans based on testing and diagnostics that examine the body's weaknesses and strengths.

After four decades working with the most knowledgeable experts in every field, I've been able to put together practices, protocols, and products—all of which will get you better sooner rather than later and may save your life. In recent times, these are the practices that shaped my recovery from long Covid and brought me back from the brink. I'm sharing my knowledge from every angle BUT everything pivots on how much effort you're going to put in. Think of it this way: *no effort, no result.*

I have focused on the ideal ways to reduce stress, improve brain performance, stay fit, improve immunity, and create healthy sleep habits. My clinic and medical associates were early advocates of the testing methodology of comprehensive blood work and genetic testing before it gained popularity. My network includes elite doctors—cardiologists, endocrinologists, neurologists, gynecologists, and various other specialists—who work alongside me and my clients, bringing a stable community and team.

My clients look for the most relevant information to amplify their performance at any level. Many of them are high functioning and travel extensively through international time zones, but have poor eating habits, don't know how to sleep, and may not be at their best. Most people who contact me are well aware of my years working in the functional health field. I've authored four books on personalized nutrition, tactics for life extension, dietary eating guidelines for children, and exceptional care for people as they move through all stages of their life. Even though I believed I was prepared for practically any illness that I could have faced, Covid proved me wrong. Covid was not a practical viability—but it is real and has taken over my life and the lives of many others. It can punish you if you are not prepared for its complexities.

Full recovery from long Covid, let alone recovery at all, is not a walk in the park for most people, especially those with preexisting health conditions or past a certain age. Many of those people will suffer the consequences of long Covid for months and even years. You may feel fine, but the virus may have laid down land mines that remain dormant, quietly wreaking havoc in your body. In an indefinite time later, in some spare moment of diminished immunity, it could rear its ugly head and capitalize on an unsuspecting body.

No one, not even top epidemiologists or the CDC, knows what is coming down the pike with this rapidly mutating virus. No one can predict what might occur. No one can predict what might happen when the virus attacks—and attack it does. For those who believe they have "natural immunity," that they somehow will not get it or won't suffer, think again. The Omicron and other variants have and will take over transmissions—the virus changes the playing field rapidly and may render neutral what worked with the Delta variant, or even the original variant.

I would know—I *was* one of those people who believed in natural immunity. I was naive enough to believe that over forty years of intense routine and regulation would spare me from a global health crisis—*but I was wrong*. Even those who drink green juice daily, or participate in Ironman triathlons, or have a young and potent immune system—you may have to deal with this too.

I was the healthiest version of myself I could possibly have been. I went in for elective neck surgery and it simply did not occur to me that I'd come out with Covid and that Covid would nearly kill me.

Vaccines were not available at the time. I certainly believe that if I had been vaccinated, I would not have nearly died. But since I had not yet received the vaccine, I know I would not have survived if not for my years of training as a health practitioner and my disciplined care of my own body. If I had not been dedicated to staying healthy and following these protocols, I would have been overcome by long Covid.

I believe anyone can fight a valiant battle against the issues that this deadly virus can create if one is disciplined. Preparing oneself for the harm it may cause is essential, if and when one is infected, with or without a vaccine.

PROTOCOL 1

Sleep: The Magic Ingredient

Sleep is an essential ingredient to being strong at any age, immunologically or otherwise. Mastering the art of sleep is usually the first step I recommend to my clients before any other treatment or routines are put in place. Although I had been actively tweaking and working on a perfect routine for my own sleep, Covid nonetheless absolutely shattered my work. If the regulation of one's sleep is capricious before Covid, then the virus might be even more disruptive. Since the early days of the virus, there have been a host of studies that have shown the benefits of sleep specifically during the critical period of recovery from any number of illnesses, due to the problems that pathogenic immunological attacks cause on the body.

Recovering from Covid revolves around diligently planning to fight exhaustion. The key is seeking out *reparative sleep.* In the weeks and months of discomfort that may follow, sleep cannot just be a respite from the various side effects of the illness, but rather a tool in fighting them off and eventually defeating them.

As I chronicled earlier, I could barely sleep during my extended hospitalization. Beyond my own bodily discomfort, the combination of constant blaring light, periodic wake-ups to check my oxygen levels, and the cries of anguish from my fellow patients throughout my hospital room kept me awake.

Returning home, suffering from immense sleep deprivation, I struggled to find a way to get any rest at all. I knew there had to be a master plan for restorative sleep, so I got to work putting together a sleep "cocktail." Let me explain that the nutraceuticals included are substances that physiologically help against chronic disease, provide biological and health benefits, and come from food-based products. In other words, nutraceuticals provide many beneficial effects against health problems, not just Covid, and were vital in my fight to sleep again. In combination with certain peptides and nootropics, I found relief.

I am offering you all the supplements I have studied and used myself to induce sleep, extend sleep time, reduce abrupt wake-ups, and engender fresh, full rest. These properties are not intended to narcotize you to sleep, but rather give you the high-quality sleep that likely has been disrupted because of viral damage to circadian rhythms—they can also normalize natural melatonin levels within the brain. Because I was suffering from a post-traumatic stress disorder caused by both the virus and hospital stay, I was desperate to try any of the nutraceuticals and supplements that might work. I experimented with some alone and some in combination. I also do not take chances with clients suffering from sleep deprivation, and when I have a client who comes to me with sleep problems, I ask them to monitor the supplements—**there is no one rule by which everyone must abide**. For example, although melatonin is a household name, and a typical over-the-counter sleep aid, people still respond to it differently. Given in small amounts, melatonin may improve some of the sleep disturbances resulting from the viral infection. There are doctors who prescribe very high amounts, but I don't agree with them. Personally, Melatonin makes me sleep well but enervates me when I'm awake. I always recommend starting with the lowest doses and increase or decrease while monitoring the results.

I know the supplements that work, and when combined, depending on the person and their sensitivity, they will improve sleep. Some of these may make you go into a deep sleep quickly, some might extend the amount of time to sleep without waking, and some will improve REM and deep sleep. All of these supplements allow the body to get the sleep it requires so the immune system can repair itself and you can wake up well rested.

While many of these products may be unfamiliar, they can each serve in the fight against exhaustion and the battle to find restorative sleep. Each one works on different parts of the brain to help it quiet down and allow better sleep. In the chapter on nutraceuticals and supplements, I cover the various products and combinations to normalize sleep patterns and circadian rhythms.

Routines are incredibly important for good sleep as well. I try to go to sleep at approximately the same time each night and wake up and get out of bed at the same time each morning, regardless of how I feel. With a good night's sleep, morning routines are recognized, within neuroscientific and biological circles, as crucial to setting up your day and feeling healthy and alert.

To improve my sleep, I also meditate and use different meditation techniques and tools. Hours before bed I do a guided meditation and I use a specific pair of headphones that aid my sleep goals. Good sleep involves quieting any distracting voices inside, voices that originate from not only the virus, but also any residual difficulty in your life that may have been impacted by your illness.

And I needed these tools, because I needed sleep. The voices in my head droned endlessly following my hospital stint. My entire brain, and the coping mechanisms I had developed in my adult life, had no answer for Covid. I experienced a great deregulation. Again, the traumatic events of the depths of Covid had fully penetrated my blood-brain barrier, and had ignited an amygdala hijack. I had been subject to terrible conditions in the hospital, coupled with the chronic pain and anxiety surrounding the virus itself, and once the hospital discharged me, I had no idea how to begin quieting the voices, or really how to begin anything in order to feel better. It felt impossible to be the person I had been before. The traumatic stressors directly impacted my sleep. One or two errant thoughts could have my mind racing for hours. The root of trauma, in general, comes from ruminating on the past and being preoccupied with the future. Covid stripped me of the ability to mitigate those fears and worries. At that point, I actually had something tangible and unhelpable to ruminate on. Something ominous and uncertain to fear. It took me back to square one, and I tried everything to fix it. I cannot say that it has subsided completely, but I am far better than I had been.

I also include other sleep and meditation-inducing devices in greater detail later on.

PROTOCOL 2

Rebuilding the Body (and Immune System)

As I mentioned earlier, my clients and friends often ask me: "How can I live longer and remain free from infirmity?" which I interpret as, "How do I expand my well-being as I get older?" As humans age, there is a well-documented decline in general functionality as the body begins to accrue certain infirmities and mutations. Heart disease, diabetes, and dementia are just a few that come to mind, but in truth there is an innumerable amount of ailments that can attack the body as it ages. Over time, depending on any given person's genetics, there may exist a predisposition toward certain diseases. Given contemporary scientific advancement, genetics can be tested and a person can prepare for the infirmities to which they may be more susceptible as they get older, which I always recommend to my clients. Age wears down white blood cells in the body, making them less efficient than when we were younger.

All of this is to say that we all want to keep our immune systems up to date, working on developing a robust response that can effectively halt any disruption. Because we do many things that damage the immune system, we need to build back our health and make it behave properly, for when that time may come.

Now, although this is not as practice-based as the other protocols here, I knew while in the pit of despair how much worse off I would have been without even some preparation. This section is more about the gravity of importance as opposed to delineating practice-based information. The process of strengthening the immune system is the number one thing that anyone can do to avoid serious or long effects from Covid or other viral infections—though my preparation for immunity certainly was not potent enough. Regardless, I have always taken my clients over this hurdle at different stages in my work. One part of immune system strength comes from prebiotics, probiotics, amino acids, and more. It also comes from good, measured sleep, as well as breathing exercises and lung expansion. All of these things have some measurable impact on the health of the immune system. A powerful immune system is a beneficial asset and aspect of a functional, working body. Many of the people who suffer from long Covid, even those who are vaccinated, were unhealthy people prior to their diagnosis.

What I have worked on is developing practices, habits, and products that make every immune system work with greater vigor. It does not matter whether someone has had Covid, or is suffering from long Covid. These practices are intended to prepare for the worst, to withstand any onslaught that may come with the virus or otherwise.

As I mentioned in the beginning of this part of the book, the availability of vaccination has been an essential advance in preparedness. Vaccination became widely available just two weeks after my neck operation—I suffered hugely without this boon, which has undoubtedly saved countless lives. Without it, I almost died, and I was very healthy going into that operation.

But, in the end, despite vaccination, powerful mutations of the virus have proven to break through. Nonetheless, there is an exponentially greater chance of survival with the vaccine, even if great illness strikes.

I will start with the basics. It is important to dedicate oneself, as I did myself, to the following rudimentary protocols before continuing on to the more comprehensive protocols, as well as the probiotics, prebiotics, peptides, nootropics, nutraceuticals, and more that I cover in the following chapters. These will provide the armor necessary to battle this monster virus and all of its potential mutations to date.

PROTOCOL 3
The Paleo/Ketogenic Diet

In the wake of my hospital stint, a thirty-five-pound weight loss had left me a mere shadow of my former self. I was already lean, having been a longtime a marathon runner, but Covid left my body in crisis mode. Repairing the body and immune system requires a strict diet that addresses weight and muscle loss, loss of taste and smell, and other side effects that may have occurred. Most people, specifically in America, eat a suboptimal diet that adds nothing but calories and carbs, along with low functionality. The usual craveable foods, high in excess processed fats and sugar, are useless for recovery—in fact, they usually aid in deteriorating the body further. Clients often tell me that they are unsure they can push through on a strict eating plan, to which I say, "What do you propose to do?"

There were two diet structures that appealed to me most. I have recommended both to clients and friends in the past, though I had not participated in the diets, mostly because my usual diet is both rigid and highly optimized to fit my lifestyle. The first style of eating was a paleo diet. I have said several times how I knew that I needed to get back to basics in order to give my body a hard reset, and there is no greater diet regression plan than one that harkens back to the Paleolithic era. The paleo diet insists on foods that, in a previous era, could have been obtained by the primal method of hunting and gathering. These foods consist of lean meat, seafood, fruits, vegetables, nuts, seeds, and berries. Some of the draws of a paleo diet include better blood pressure control, improvement of cardiovascular risk factors, improvement of liver health, and the absolute shunning of processed foods.

I created a hybrid plan, partnering the paleo aspect with the well-known ketogenic diet. Keto is based on low-carb and high-fat eating. I needed healthy fats more than anything in the early stages of my recovery.

The high fat content meant that the fats themselves would be converted to energy, of which I was lacking tremendously. I could use the fat I was consuming to make energy in order to do even the smallest of tasks that required all of my willpower to achieve. I had such little energy that every bit that I could acquire would help. Along with intermittent fasting, which I will discuss shortly, I could achieve a state of ketosis to adequately transfer fats to energy as quickly as possible.

There have even been studies conducted at this point that have promoted the ketogenic diet as a substantial and helpful aid to recovery from Covid symptoms, especially those that may linger beyond the ten-to-fourteen-day ailment window. Ketones provided by the ketogenic diet can indeed target complications from respiratory issues and viruses alike, especially in patients who are either obese or have health complications that may make recovery more difficult. The ketogenic diet can also aid in a post-rehabilitation lifestyle change that can work to prevent complications for future viral infections or whatever may be coming down the pipeline for this pandemic or future health risks. This is especially helpful if the patient is unvaccinated.

Of course, both keto and paleo have added benefits that were beyond the scope of my recovery, the most prevalent being weight loss. I did not need to lose weight; I needed to gain it back. However, weight loss may be a part of your journey, whether directly after Covid or in later stages of your recovery, and in that sense this diet can provide a helping hand.

My diet plan in toto is not entirely beginner friendly, but I would certainly not be opposed to someone taking it day by day. Each day, I urge you to try to be 1 percent better than the last. Creating this protocol became therapeutic for me at my worst, researching which foods I could eat to gain back the strength I lost, envisioning the specific flavors that I could not taste at that moment. By the time I had finished planning and began to follow the guidelines, they helped immensely in reducing my anguish. I slowly began to regain my weight and energy, instead of lingering in bed and giving in to the natural compulsion to eat poorly, either looking for a quick hit of lost dopamine or out of sheer apathy

Before dealing with any diet plan, I always urge my clients to get a full workup from their doctor. Diagnostics and blood work can show what else might have been affected by Covid, and these findings may reveal medical issues that could affect the direction of any recovery program.

After Covid, I received a complete cardiological examination, physical examination, and comprehensive blood tests to check for inflammatory markers and beyond. I also had several consultations with my regular pulmonologist to determine the current status of my lungs and address any breathing concerns. This is a routine I have since maintained as well, and I am more vigilant of these visits than I had been before Covid.

I found out that my kidney and renal function had dropped by about 30 percent and my blood urea changed dramatically as well. I had also developed anemia as a result of the virus. All of these appointments later factored into my diet, as I had to deal with new deficiencies due to Covid.

They also found that, in the hospital, my blood pressure rose to an extremely high, perilous level. I breached a cataclysmic 230, and the remedy that they had fed me, high blood pressure medication, only made it worse in recovery. After a few weeks, however, they did not find anything too dangerous in my blood work, and that reinforced my decision to go on a high-fat diet with a lot of animal protein. I knew it was a huge risk to do this, but it was also a risk I had to take. I needed any additional energy and cushioning on my body that I could obtain.

Once I finished that high-fat diet section of my recovery, I began reintroducing elements of my previous diet, one with Greek and Mediterranean influences, plant-based foods, heavy in seafood and vegetables. I began to enjoy what I was eating once again. It was improving the quality of my health, and preventing any more stress on my heart and internal organs. That combination was the exact purpose behind the paleo and ketogenic diets I had been employing. I was hacking my body and getting my muscle back.

Covid decimated several parts of my body, those I had worked hard on to secure from distress. After I was released from the hospital, I developed a terrific pain in my stomach, which turned out to be a rupture in my bowel. I was in enormous pain and began to bleed internally. After a CAT scan revealed an infection in my bowel, I had yet another reason to build back my body, this time my stomach, bowels, and colon. I knew how essential it was—70 percent of immune system function is determined by the bacteria in your bowel. It also regulates a substantial amount of mental activity and moods, pivoting off the brain/gut axis.

The bowel system regulates a myriad of bodily functions—white blood cell efficacy, brain power, state of mind, clarity of thought, anxiety management—which are essential to long Covid recovery and beyond.

Returning home from three weeks of various drugs and substandard food, all of the good bacteria (my microbiome) throughout my body had been decimated. I needed a plan to rebuild it.

My plan included a highly dynamic diet, one that differed from my normal eating ritual. I had to add foods and drinks to build back muscle and exclude those that kept me lean. The goal was to create a diet that had a high degree of functionality to build power, energy, and my microbiome, and one that could provide the nutrients to help my immune system work better and protect my brain function.

My initial diet included an eating plan to gain back weight quickly. Although hardly a rabid carnivore in my pre-Covid days, I followed a paleo/carnivore plan, eating meat three times a day. I had experience with the paleo diet, mostly as a plan I had recommended to deeply exhausted clients as a way to naturally rebuild energy. Paleo was central to improvement, adding calories and rebuilding my muscles. My meals consisted of a lot of fat and little starch. I was on a mission to eat my way to normalcy.

Even though a paleo diet was helpful for weight and muscle gain, it comes with its own challenges, one of which is constipation. This is where I began implementing prebiotics into my diet, little by little, in order to offset any issues with recovery. I will be going into more detail in later sections about the specifics. Again, every detail of the diet, and each supplement I introduced, came from a place of *regeneration*, as I needed to rebuild my microbiome.

Even today, as I have gotten as close as possible to my pre-Covid self, I continue the same regimen, with modifications after I have regained my muscle. The regimen includes prebiotics, a smoothie, and multiple supplements and nutraceuticals. In fact, throughout the day, I take about a hundred different pills—but this is not necessary for everyone, and certainly not for someone who has no experience with functional medicine practice. I only crafted my supplement protocol after consultation with several authorities, all of which knew the projected impact of each supplement and how it may accelerate my path out from long Covid.

Once I regained the weight I had lost, I returned to my pre-Covid diet which relied heavily on plant-based food and complex carbohydrates. These cuisines rely heavily on plant-based food and complex carbohydrates. I stopped eating meat for the most part, instead replacing it with healthy fats—my go-to has always been olive oil. I eliminated as much as possible from the typical Western diet, spurning processed foods, sugar, and alcohol. I drink very minimal coffee. I encourage these food guidelines for the first few months, though the guidelines can be expanded after a few months.

An error I often see my clients make is wanting to count calories. People perceive hyperspecificity as a helpful tool in losing weight or maintaining a healthy body. In my experience, it is much more likely for it to hinder recovery. I find that counting calories becomes a worthwhile distraction, a mirage of health, that can make people obey a calorie-counter before they would listen to their own body. My trick is to teach people to become **instinctual eaters**, and take note of what their body says, not what the calorie or fat content number may indicate. A healthy lifestyle is about anything but the numbers. So women's and fitness magazines that only focus on the numbers are of no use or consequence to me. When you are in touch with overall healthier practices and take your body seriously, counting calories becomes irrelevant. I can delineate the foods and drinks that help in vague categories, and how they may come together and work in tandem, but the amount of these foods and drinks to consume is up to your own personal discretion. Literally, **trust your gut**.

Something important to note is that I practiced **intermittent fasting** once I gained the majority of my weight back. I had practiced it quite often before Covid, but I found that once I started gaining some muscle back, it proved to be incredibly useful as a recovery tool. Intermittent fasting gives the body a complete break from digesting food continually.

As humans, the more energy that comes into our bodies, the closer we are to our eventual demise. In direct opposition of American eating culture, the one that literally hinges on shoving food down your throat, intermittent fasting shows the importance of undereating, which is built into the human body by nature.

There once was a time where we were foraging and gathering, and at that time in human history, meats, protein, and most sturdy and substantial food was uncertain. There was no guarantee that anyone would be able to consume protein for days, sometimes weeks, on end. We were forced to eat intermittently as a consequence of our nature.

Fasting pairs well with something like a paleo diet— the truest reset possible within the scope of our bodies. It can improve hearing, vision, and can potentially affect smell capacity as well. These are the sort of things that happen when predators in the animal community need help to find their prey. It is a natural response for a dominant organism. The capacity for hunting improves, and this has been lost in humans as sustenance has become so accessible.

In a culture of instant gratification and boundless consumption, we have built habits to eat immediately and all the time. The foods that we are bound to eat are highly processed and produced with chemicals to make you want to eat more, which leads to overeating and a culture of obesity. Intermittent fasting also makes you get more out of your organs, since they do not have to be constantly breaking food down. The liver, somach, gut, gallbladder, and many more can now provide their most useful and base functions without the added pressure of digestion.

Fasting can also have both a soothing and calming effect on the body. It encourages deeper and better sleep, waking up lighter, and a better mood overall throughout the day. It also affects several aspects of the immune system, aspects that may have been altered dramatically through Covid. It can increase certain enzymes in the body that are self-repairing, like the processes of apoptosis or autophagy. Though autophagy can still be achieved with certain supplements, it is easier and more efficient to fast in order to gain natural benefits.

So I knew I needed to start fasting then, given the tremendous and damaging impact on my body, an impact that I could not even know for certain, at the time, but I just had a hunch. I assumed based on that feeling and experience in this field that I had aged my body substantially. In addition to the fasting itself, there are also peptides that can have an effect like this on the body.

This diet is even more essential if you are overweight or clinically obese. Your body demands high consumption of protein and vegetables, no starch, and no alcohol. In case you need to consume something sweet, I recommend stevia or monk fruit. Based on preliminary statistics, your chances of getting Covid and dying are exponentially higher if you are overweight, have type 2 diabetes, or are living with a preexisting health condition, certainly a chronic heart-related illness. If your percentage of body fat is above 26 percent then you must do this if you want to build a more resilient body. You could also be saving your life.

THE DIET ITSELF

Weight Gain

ANIMAL PROTEIN: It had been many years since I had needed to rely on animal protein. My protein has come in plant-based forms most of my adult life, as well as in the supplements I take for digestion and gut health. Additionally, I found that fatty fish and seafood could tide my body over for the protein I needed. But my new task was weight gain. Animal protein would be the quickest way to regain muscle mass and fat in general. Extremely high consumption of animal proteins would provide me with all of the essential amino acids I needed, while simultaneously adding much-needed support for my weary bones. I could also offset some of the issues with a high-volume animal protein diet with the other parts of my diet, as well as my prebiotics, which would sustain a steady intake of good bacteria. The risk was still great given the damage Covid had potentially done to some of my internal organs. But the risk paid off.

LOW-GLYCEMIC FRUIT: I had to keep my blood sugar low while recovering, but I still needed energy from my food. I chose to load up on low-glycemic fruit to maximize the carbohydrate levels while also maintaining a healthy blood sugar level in recovery. I needed to make sure that the fruits I ate would not damage my body further, or hinder me in some other way to make my recovery more difficult. Low-glycemic fruit induces better metabolism, so the food I was eating could fuel me faster and most efficiently. While this was never a centerpiece of my meals, it was a frequent addition to my carnivorous diet in order to provide fibrous carbohydrates.

HEALTHY FATS: Healthy fats aid in heart health and lower bad cholesterol levels. I needed a mass amount of the fatty acids that my body could not produce on its own. The healthy fats I ate were found in butter, olive oil, sesame oil, coconut oil, artisanal cheeses, eggs, coconut milk yogurt, almond milk yogurt, oat milk yogurt, goat's milk yogurt, and full-fat cow's milk yogurt. There are options with or without dairy, so do not let that be a barrier for consuming important fats.

After Weight Gain

Once I had gained the weight back, I reintroduced a large amount of the food I had eaten before, as well as an ample amount of starches. I ate mostly yams, squash, beans, rice, and quinoa—plus a lot of seafood. In terms of my vegetable intake, I now needed high cruciferous vegetables, mainly broccoli, kale, cabbage, Swiss chard, spinach, dandelion, and arugula. Cruciferous vegetables, or "super vegetables," contain high fiber, vitamins, minerals, and phytochemicals, and are generally the best vegetables for your health. I only could introduce them now because my stomach was stronger and I could handle it.

SAMPLE DIET FOR WEIGHT GAIN

BREAKFAST: One medium to large flank steak, two hard-boiled eggs, steamed vegetables

LUNCH: Large filet of grilled salmon, roasted vegetables, cooked with ample amount of olive oil, two handfuls of mixed nuts

SNACK: Coconut yogurt with mixed berries, cashew milk yogurt

DINNER: Roast chicken, roasted vegetables

SAMPLE DIET AFTER WEIGHT GAIN

Remember, I ate this while practicing intermittent fasting.

BREAKFAST: Morning smoothie, gluten-free tortilla with scrambled eggs and chopped vegetables OR vegetable omelet with salmon or sardines, cup of coconut/almond milk yogurt with mixed berries

LUNCH: 8–10 oz. salmon with rice or quinoa, roasted vegetables (usually a combination of cruciferous vegetables like broccoli, kale, cauliflower, and carrots), half of an avocado, sprinkled with nuts

DINNER: Chicken or lamb with rice or quinoa, roasted vegetables

DESSERT: Gluten-free and sugar-free cookies OR 70 percent cacao dark chocolate OR almond milk / coconut milk yogurt with dark chocolate, berries, and nuts

PROTOCOL 4

Routine, Routine, Routine

My arduous return to health necessitated adherence to a daily schedule. It might appear to be closer to a ritual than a routine, but it became pivotal not only for my physical progression, but also my mental health. I remembered how important it became to me in the hospital to plan this routine at all. It was an escape—a fantasy that could be fulfilled if I ever got out. Once I did, I made good to my withered self. I knew I needed to have a plan and stick with it if I wanted to recuperate.

From what my fellow long Covid sufferers have told me, one's appetite for living diminishes tremendously through a long and often uncertain recovery timetable. Even though I felt totally knocked out and down, I never gave in to lethargy, since some studies have indicated that dementia can be an additional residual of Covid, and brain cells may also be damaged.

Prior to Covid, my morning routine usually never took longer than an hour. My new life required four hours of focused effort. This is what it looked like.

Ice Baths: As I began to get my strength back, I discovered the value of ice baths. The healing effects of ice baths are well documented, as many athletes take them after long stretches of physical activity. My ice baths reduced the pain in my body caused by my chronic aching, as well as reducing inflammation. Additionally, they were beyond powerful in helping me secrete dopamine in order to clear my brain fog. My neural regeneration improved dramatically with the help of ice baths.

Breathing Exercises: Next, I followed up my ice baths with breathing exercises. I have used several breathing devices in the past, but I mostly had to learn to use new and different devices to help me expand my lungs and increase my lung capacity to what it had been before, because in those early weeks I could hardly breathe at all. I used a device designed for athletes called The Breather to make my lungs work harder and increase their strength. One of my favorites is the Airofit Breathing Trainer, which is even more advanced and intense, but I will include more on the devices themselves later. My breathing journey centered around deep breathing. I used yoga and exercises to build up my lung capacity and transmit oxygen from my lungs to the peripheral places in my body that needed it, like my limbs, muscles, and brain as well. I would practice a daily routine, looking to improve it incrementally, no matter how hard it was on my body. There were days where

I would feel like passing out from the exertion. And yet, in spite of the difficulty at first, I did indeed improve daily until I could wean myself off of the home oxygen tank, and breathe freely without being winded.

Whether or not you have had a version of Covid with pneumonic symptoms, your lungs may still be compromised. Doctors are now slowly catching on to post-Covid rehabilitation, which begins with learning breathing techniques to normalize blood gasses and sequester carbon dioxide, for its relaxing and anti-anxiety-producing effects. These breathing exercises and devices are essential regardless of the severity of your illness because, undoubtedly, your lungs have been affected in some way.

A Bloomberg *Prognosis* podcast from late 2021 cited a study being conducted at New York's Mount Sinai Health System, which claims that it takes "easily" 100 days of slowly conditioning the autonomic nervous system so it gets used to being challenged." I encourage anyone who was hit with Covid pneumonia to invest in any of the breathing devices that I list in the Additional Therapies section, because they are crucial to building and rebuilding lung capacity, which is central to recovering your health at large. These devices and exercises are much more effective and advanced than the ones suggested in the Mount Sinai long Covid program being offered at the moment.

Gratitude Meditation: Gratitude was an ineffably salient element of my life that entered and quickly blossomed in my Covid recovery. To work on my mindfulness daily, I really favor *Waking Up with Sam Harris* for a multitude of reasons, including being able to focus my mind, instead of feeling it drift away, which can happen with other mindfulness practices. This app has several mini-apps within it; besides the mental benefits that I derive from it, the app gave me a solid platform on which to think about my condition and potential remedies. On my best days, *Waking Up* allowed me to think more clearly, with greater rigor about the road ahead and the new direction my life had taken. On a bad day, I could seek refuge in a calming place instead of beating myself up over my condition and deteriorating sense of self.

I will continue to extol the virtues of *Waking Up* as long as I use it. I cannot overstate its impact, though it was not the only type of gratitude I practiced daily. I also used a gratitude journal that I would write in every day. I would usually write in it once in the morning and once in the evening. It was a terrific tool for letting go of the negativity related to long Covid and focusing on what I did have, and how I was grateful to even be alive. Journaling became as important to my routine as anything in this book.

Exercise: I stretched and exercised every morning because my body is tight after such a long gap in my running regimen. Remember, in order to regain my strength and flexibility, I took many of my cues from Clear's book, *Atomic Habits*, and began to form new habits, doing a little bit more each day. When I began moving my body more and began exercising, looking to regain my favorite outlet, I would often feel tired prematurely, frustrated with my inability to function. I no longer had the strength I used to, and in the early stages I would power through the pain regardless, often through tears. It started when I began doing my daily push-ups. It may seem like a banal exercise compared to the influx of classes and fad workouts of today, but it was the only thing I could do. It was the only power I had in me. Once I had the ability to even get myself out of bed, which was an endeavor in itself, I began with one push-up; the next day, I tried two. It would not take much for me to lose all of my energy, to collapse in exhaustion. But I kept at it.

Breathing itself was an exercise for my depleted body. I would pick up the Airofit device and attempt to do a ten- or fifteen-minute session, a few times a day. I put it on the hardest difficulty—if I could not function at an advanced level, I did not want to function at all. Even after a short session, I would be soaked in sweat and drained.

After I could move a bit better, I ordered resistance bands, as I lacked stability in my movement and wanted a diversity of training given as little of the world I could access at the time. I would use the bands for intense workouts, usually high intensity interval training (HIIT). When I started with the bands, I would use the easiest ones, which might have been the resistance strength made for a small child—but I had to start somewhere. I would be exhausted after five or ten minutes. Do you see the pattern? Almost immediate exhaustion and my body giving out on me, often and quickly. But the through line across these workouts and routines was willpower, and my eventual return to strength. The last at-home workout I tried to accomplish was the TRX Home System. I wanted to try to hold up my own body weight. I got the hang of it eventually, after some trials, as I was several weeks into strength training.

Lastly, somewhat related to my exercise routine was my bodywork. I would have a deep tissue massage, once or twice a week. The sessions would be one or two hours and were critical to removing inflammation. They would knock me out to sleep on the nights I had them.

There's power in making tiny gains, and you can either get 1 percent better or 1 percent worse each day. There is no telling whether an incremental difference will impact you much today, or perhaps even tomorrow. But as time goes on, these small improvements or declines compound. I have found, not just with myself but with my clients, that there is a substantial gap between people who make slightly better decisions on a daily basis and those who choose not to. Everything I told myself then was to save my ass, and I'm still telling myself the same stuff every day for that same reason.

Focus on Yourself and Your Improvement: There have been rapid studies that have shown even five minutes of bad news can affect thinking for the whole day and, in practice, ruin a day from the start. For the most part, during the healing process, I needed to protect myself from exposure to bad news. It was toxic, and slithered its way into my brain, subtly cutting off thoughts of self-improvement. In fact, though I hate to admit this, I was emotionally apathetic early in my recovery, and had very little desire or motivation to do anything.

Listening to the news only made it worse. Both my phone and social media aggravated this problem even further. Curtailing my time paying attention to bad news and my general mindlessness opened up a great deal of time to start writing again and falling back in love with reading. It may sound cliché, but both mass media and social media exist to make you feel worse about yourself. It is an active choice to decide to better yourself on a daily basis, and prioritize your sanity over the minor, counterfeit dopamine that these outlets provide.

5

Your Survival Kit

I have openly shared my experiences, which were nothing less than a matter of life and death. Due to the revelatory nature of my illness, and the work I have done to fix what had been broken, my new, current client base includes Covid and post-Covid sufferers willing to do almost anything to feel better. Through this experience, I can comfortably say that I know exactly how they feel. It is easy for me to empathize, be compassionate, and share what I have learned and practiced. Previously, at the start of my illness, I worried about what would happen to my clientele as a cause of my illness. But, because of the hardship I overcame, I now have more tools to engage with my professional life, beyond my previous concerns. This would not have happened without the plan that I devised and enacted at my lowest point of long Covid.

Doctors have been giving out traditional medicine to Covid patients and sufferers, but there just clearly has not been an efficacious enough strategy to curb future symptoms of the virus, as well as those dreadful aftershocks that seem to appear with great frequency. In fact, if Covid patients only adhere to what their medical providers make available in the wake of their illness, I have real doubts about whether they can improve. This is such a new virus, and the traditional method has not been outlined strongly enough. I, for one, experienced this—I know what got me out of the hospital, and out of my recovery bed.

In the twenty-first century, there has been a rapid, global development surrounding a whole new field of nutrients, vitamins, minerals, amino acids, herbs, and oils, which I collectively refer to as nutraceuticals. In addition, there are magnificent peptides and nootropics that have been researched and developed, many of which I have recommended to my clients or taken myself in my lifetime. These supplements can be considered an arsenal for recuperation, weapons to rebuild an immune system that has taken both unseen and unforeseen damage. Even without Covid, remember, I recommend building the body's armor in order to handle whatever virus or illness comes to prevalence.

What must be understood, first and foremost, is that nutraceuticals are *not* prescription drugs that a doctor might order. For the most part, they are food-based compounds of enormous benefit in helping strengthen the immune system and can be considered alternatives to pharmaceutical products. The other categories of peptides and nootropics are equally sound. Since the dawn of the Covid era, both epidemiologists and biostatisticians not only expect the Covid virus to be able to reinfect former patients in the next few years, but also predict other factors, pandemic or not, may threaten our immune systems in the near future as well.

Tossing down a daily vitamin C, with a handful of other random pills and multivitamins, might seem like it will bolster the immune system adequately—in my opinion, this approach is not enough. The most threatening aspects of this virus and any future immune-targeting illness require a far more sophisticated and targeted plan. All of the products I recommend have been vetted by me personally. Some of them have been used for thousands of years across the world. Many of them have been validated by the scientific community, as well.

I recommend prebiotics and probiotics because building (or rebuilding) the gut microbiome is crucial. What goes on inside that organ regulates 70 percent or more of the body's immune system response. My plan includes a broad family of probiotics and fermented foods, a highly functional diet with no processed foods, little or no alcohol consumption, and eight hours of high-quality sleep daily. To bolster and modulate the immune system, I have added supplements and carefully chosen pre- and probiotics to address the individual's needs.

The nootropics, peptides, and nutraceuticals are equally important. I have researched and put all of these supplements into practice, and they can absolutely improve the body's response to a brain, gut, and immune system disaster like Covid or long Covid.

Also, I do encourage IV vitamin therapy for my clients, which, if carefully formulated by a trained practitioner, can have multiple fortifying effects including improved brain function, exercise performance, anti-inflammation, anti-aging, and benefits of strengthening the immune system.

As I have said before, I design the combinations based on the individual's needs, but my medical team oversees the various supplements and administers the IVs. These formulas have been crafted over my forty years of practice and are combinations of compounded nutrients that range all the way from the highest doses of vitamin C to specific minerals, nootropics, antioxidants, and peptides. I am sharing my winning protocols and products and again ask that you consult with your physician or functional practitioner in tandem with this guide.

In recommending these products, it all comes down to personal programming and seeing what works best. Not all of these supplements should be taken at once, and certainly not immediately. It behooves the newcomer to start slowly and ramp up with more comfort, if at all.

I also have included additional therapies, products, devices, books, apps, and more in this book to further demonstrate the variety of resources available to those struggling with long Covid.

PROBIOTICS AND PREBIOTICS

Probiotics

Probiotics are living microorganisms that play a critical role in maintaining good health. They are present in many foods, but are often destroyed by heat processing. These live probiotic cultures populate the intestinal tract where they play a key role in digestive and immune system health. Probiotics are live bacteria—but this is good bacteria, and it has great health benefits. Proper digestion is essential for the body to absorb and utilize the nutrients it needs. Seventy-five percent of the cells necessary for the immune system can also have a profound beneficial effect on brain function, which is effectively connected to the gastrointestinal tract.

I sought out probiotics because of the deregulation of the axis between my brain and gut. Due to the poor quality of the hospital food, as well as the damage that Covid inflicted on my bowels, I needed a combination of probiotics that would help set me on track. I had to counteract all of the bad bacteria I had accumulated in my body with good bacteria that would act as a buffer for my body in its recovery.

When it comes to probiotics, I did already have some that I had previously used on a daily basis. But I had to get creative in a place of rebuilding. These are my preferred probiotic supplements:

Immune system: A general probiotic supplement that can help rebuild the immune system, specifically rebuilding upper respiratory tract health. The product I recommend is **HMF Immune** from **Genestra**.

General Gut Health Probiotic: The benefits of a catchall probiotic are general intestinal health, natural immune response, regularity of bowel movements, and aid in digesting lactose and other hard-to-digest foods. The three products I recommend are **Primal Defense Ultra** from **Garden of Life** and **ProBioMax DF** and **ProBioMax 350** from **Xymogen**.

Lactobacillus Plantarum: A probiotic that operates like a brain/gut regulator and improves mood. It also promotes general gut health and controls bloating and gas in the digestive tract. The product I recommend is **Solace**.

Prebiotics

Often paired with probiotics, prebiotics are compounds in food that encourage the growth of beneficial microorganisms. The best example is their use in the gastrointestinal tract, where prebiotics can change the composition of organisms in the gut microbiome. These typically non-digestible fiber compounds pass undigested through the upper part of the GI tract and stimulate growth of the good bacteria that inhabit the large bowel. Like probiotics, they are considered functional food components somewhere between food and drugs.

Prebiotics work in tandem with probiotics. While probiotics promote beneficial bacteria growth in the gut, prebiotic foods and carbs are incredibly fibrous.

The bacteria produced by the probiotics consume the fibrous prebiotics and this can lead to healthier bowel movement and intestinal health. Prebiotics exist in many foods already, like onions, bananas, and Jerusalem artichokes. But I find that isolating and stimulating prebiotic intake directly had more of a direct impact on my digestive system.

I prefer to ingest prebiotic supplements in my early morning glass of water, beverage, or smoothie. I will include more details on my morning smoothie later on. These are the prebiotics I recommend:

Flaxseed Powder: This is a powerful tool in digestive health, and I have used flaxseed powder with or without chia seed powder included. Usually the combination of the two has proven more effective for me. Both powders are extraordinary sources of fiber that improve digestion, reduce heart problems, and even promote anti-cancer protective effects. Flaxseed powder also reduces inflammation in the bowel and increases its capacity for probiotics to do their thing, adhering to the bowel walls. I use this dietary fiber prebiotic with a full glass of water to start my day in the morning. The product I recommend is **OptiFiber Lean** from **Xymogen**.

Inulin Powder: This is another type of prebiotic powder that works in conjunction with flaxseed powder. Considered a prebiotic, inulin increases the potential benefits of probiotics while additionally improving overall gut health. It can also improve episodic memory, as well as free recall. The human gut contains its own nervous system that can be disrupted and/or damaged from a multitude of challenges that go on to damage the central nervous system in the brain, thus adversely affecting the axis between the brain and the gut. Inulin can prevent damage to our gut bacteria, which I also refer to as "our second brain," and can improve both immune and brain/mood function overall. The product I recommend is **Inulin** from **It's Just**.

General Fiber Powder: Not all prebiotic supplements are specialized with certain ingredients. I recommend an over-the-top fiber supplement in addition to more specialized products in order to retain gut health and prevent constipation. I also would add that the best fiber supplements are usually gluten-free, organic, and non-GMO. The product I recommend is **Dr. Formulated Organic Prebiotic Fiber** from **Garden of Life**.

NOOTROPICS AND PEPTIDES

Nootropics

Nootropics, often referred to as "smart drugs" or cognitive enhancers, are substances that claim to improve cognitive function with an emphasis on memory, creativity, motivation, and brain performance. They can also boost attention, executive function, and mood. Some nootropics can also reduce anxiety and depression by acting on problematic and misbehaving brain centers, as well as improving quality of sleep. I had frequently used nootropics for strictly cognitive purposes pre-Covid, but I found that their effects on my mood were more prevalent after the time I had spent suffering. I knew using these specific nootropics would retrain my brain to perform at optimum levels, and would translate into better performance systemically. My mental function greatly improved with the help of nootropics.

Some nootropics are prescription based, and address conditions like attention deficit disorder, narcolepsy, and other disorders. The ones I will recommend below are all over the counter and do not require a prescription. The supplements listed below are among the ones I used.

Phenylpiracetam: This is a nootropic derivative of piracetam, which I will discuss later on. The phenyl version of this supplement aids with a general lack of focus, which is a primary symptom that I experienced with long Covid. Brain fog became a constant bulwark to productivity. The added "phenyl" in this molecule makes it more effective at passing through the blood-brain barrier, because it is fat soluble. There is even some preliminary research that suggests that phenylpiracetam can reduce depression and anxiety. The product I recommend is **Phenylpiracetam Powder** from **Nootropic Source**.

Picamilon: This is a chemical that is present in both dietary supplements and prescription drugs, though in the United States it is only available as the former. Picamilon can aid in enhancing mental alertness and athletic performance, while also benefiting those who suffer from anxiety and stress, all of which I needed. Picamilon works by breaking down in your brain into gamma-aminobutyric acid, also known as GABA, and niacin, which is a vitamin also found in many common foods. Niacin can also increase blood flow in the brain. For me, picamilon balanced my mood and restored general focus and relaxation in my body. The increase in GABA that it can stimulate greatly affected my depleted brain and improved my cerebrovascular performance as a result. The product I recommend is **Picamilon Sodium Powder** from **Nootropic source.**

Phenibut: This is another nootropic that increases GABA. Phenibut itself is actually very similar to the chemicals that exist in GABA, and it can be helpful in preventing anxiety, insomnia, and, most effectively for me after my stint in the hospital, post-traumatic stress disorder. Phenibut can be more useful in recovery than GABA itself because phenibut can cross the blood-brain barrier, while GABA cannot. Phenibut keeps a balance in your brain of GABA and glutamate, which is necessary to avoid countless brain traumas. Overall, phenibut balanced my mood, aided with mental challenges, and stimulated my dopamine receptors after such a long time with the lowest dopamine level in my adult life. The product I recommend is **Phenibut Powder** from **Nootropic Source.**

Meldonium: This is a nootropic that stimulates and enhances athletic performance. I found that meldonium primarily helped me as a way to recirculate my brain and mentally retrain myself for athletic performance. The product I recommend is **Mildronate Capsules** from **Grindeks**.

Oat Straw Extract: Oat straw is a natural, plant-based extract that can enhance cognitive performance. It can protect against brain inflammation, in part due to its unique bioactive compounds. It also aids in general cerebral circulation, as it boosts nitric oxide levels within the brain. Lastly, it can prevent anxiety and stress as well. As we age, or suffer from great illness, our dopamine naturally reduces. Oat straw is a singularly helpful tool to prevent such a drop. The product I recommend is **Oat Straw Extract** from **BulkSupplements**.

Citicoline: Usually an ingredient in nootropics I have used and experimented with in the past, citicoline has been important in my recovery for its ability to reopen dopamine centers that had been closed or damaged through my experience with the virus. It was one of the supplements I took that allowed me to look beyond my depressing circumstances and focus on the good, on my work. Citicoline has also dealt with a variety of neurological conditions centering around dysfunction, but personally I found it most helpful for increased dopamine receptors, as well as decreasing my brain fog and increasing alertness and reading comprehension and retention. The product I recommend is **Cognizin Citicoline Capsules** from **Nootropics Depot**.

Oxiracetam: An older synthetic version of a nootropic that I have used and recommended, Oxiracetam can improve memory cache and help when struggling to focus. I had a consistent, often striking, lack of concentration after Covid. Oxiracetam boosted my cognition in a serious way. While it provides a stimulatory effect, Oxiracetam does not have the notable side effects found in prescription stimulants or caffeine. It has proven to be useful for improving memory recall and cognitive function. The product I recommend is **Oxiracetam Powder** from **Nootropic Source**.

Huperzine A: This is another nootropic that improves brain function, as many of them do. Huperzine A has the additional benefit of fighting against glutamate toxicity in the brain. Remember, there must be a homeostatic relationship between GABA and glutamate levels within the brain. Huperzine A also aids in promoting short-term memory and can help with long-term brain health as you get older. It also has antioxidant properties. The product I recommend is **Huperzine A 1% Powder** from **either Nootropic Source or Nootropics Depot.**

DMAE: Also known as dimethylaminoethanol, DMAE can boost mental clarity and focus. Similar to citicoline, DMAE has a special relationship to acetylcholine. DMAE allows for more choline to be available for use in the brain, and can promote the use of acetylcholine, which promotes better concentration, memory encoding, and general cognition. DMAE can also improve mood and energy, while helping you maintain healthy sleep patterns. The product I recommend is **DMAE L-Bitartrate Powder** from **Nootropics Depot.**

Lion's Mane: This is the only nootropic I have mentioned so far that comes in the form of a mushroom. Lion's Mane has the specific benefit of stimulating the Nerve Growth Factor (NGF), which can help with depression, but more specifically, helps cognition and memory in the face of brain fog and other brain-related ailments. Lion's Mane is sometimes referred to as a "brain tonic." It can aid in brain cell regeneration, if needed. One of the primary compounds of Lion's Mane are erinacines, which can easily cross the blood-brain barrier, whose importance I have mentioned earlier. The product I recommend is **Lion's Mane** from **Primal Herb**.

Caffeine: On an extremely short-term basis, coffee can work as a minor bronchodilator, meaning that it can make breathing easier by relaxing lung muscles and widening pathways through which air can enter. Remember, I used coffee for this purpose on a very minor scale. For me, especially in the hospital, any improvement was a good improvement. I knew that if I could benefit from something even just 1 percent, I would do it, no question. I knew it could also help with the strength of my weakened liver. Coffee, in this case, however, cannot be drunk with milk and sugar—if you cannot drink it pure, then stevia and almond milk are passable alternatives. It is best used as a longevity product. Later in my recovery, and even now, I prefer matcha tea as a caffeine source, as it limits the myriad negative side effects that coffee contains, including additional stress and jitteriness, which works in direct opposition to a stable recovery. Matcha tea is a far better alternative, maintaining the bronchodilator effects that caffeine can provide, while also providing antioxidant benefits.

Peptides

Peptides are short chains of amino acids, often referred to as the "building blocks" of protein, which are linked by peptide bonds. The ones I recommend are bioactive, which means they are not necessary nutrients, but can nonetheless influence your health and recovery. By using certain peptides that actually repaired my damaged joints, I had the lenience to put off my initial surgery for at least a decade. Each peptide maximizes the efficiency and function of different systems in just the way they're designed to do. Every time a peptide enters the body, it simulates the function of a specific part of the body and will then improve its function. This process can occur regardless of whether a bodily function has deteriorated, either as a result of Covid, another physiological or biological injury, or just aging, and allows your body to operate again with greater efficiency.

Because I was so ill, I decided to experiment to see what worked. I discovered a certain family of peptides that helped my immune system and a different family of peptides that helped me gain weight—specifically completing my quest to regain *muscle* weight. I found peptides that had a major effect on my mood, alleviating my depression and anxiety, and ones that actually allowed me to recover my mental function, my focus, my alertness, and my memory—both long and short term. And because my blood pressure had risen so high as a result of Covid, which caused heart damage, I took peptides for cardiovascular repair.

In my case, peptides accelerated my recovery better than anything else. I'm going to divide the list into different categories so you can see their specific functions.

COGNITIVE IMPROVEMENT AND MOOD ENHANCEMENT

These are designated hitters for the brain, and as a result of improving brain function, systemic function often follows. Being depressed and not being able to recall things does not aid recovery. I suggest rotating these peptides on an ongoing basis during the week, since many are multi-purpose.

Cerebrolysin: A peptide focusing on nerve generation repair that can pass the blood-brain barrier and reach the neurons directly. People using cerebrolysin describe experiencing improved mental clarity, less fatigue, and better motivation. This peptide stimulates BDNF—brain-derived neurotrophic factor—encouraging the growth of brain tissue that has broken down as a consequence of aging, high stress, and illness. It is considered useful in treatments of traumatic brain injuries and stroke. This peptide is my favorite because of its great neuroregenerative powers.

Selank: This peptide works almost immediately and is often used in the treatment of anxiety and depressed moods. Selank works by directly affecting GABA neurotransmitters. By reducing neuronal excitability throughout the nervous system, Selank is helpful with improving mood.

Semax: This peptide, similar to cerebrolysin, increases BDNF, which aids in curbing anxiety and depression. Semax can also be prescribed for memory improvement, stroke, and nerve regeneration. Specifically, this peptide is best known for its neurogenic/neurorestorative properties.

HA-FGL: The "HA" part, hyaluronate, is considered "scaffolding for the brain." The "FGL" part is a sequence of amino acids critical for controlling both inflammation of the brain and cell regrowth. This peptide is a multi-hyphenate powerhouse.

Oxytocin: This peptide is hugely helpful for mood improvement. I found oxytocin contributed to my relaxation and was valuable in reducing my stress responses, including severe anxiety. Often when I would wake up at night and was unable to fall back to sleep, I would use an oxytocin nasal spray, which was one of the few things that helped me fall asleep again. Oxytocin decreases cortisol, a very important stressor and harmer.

REBUILDING ENERGY

SS-31: One of my biggest problems while recovering, and one that many long Covid sufferers experience, was tremendous fatigue. I needed to regenerate the engines within myself and stimulate my mitochondria, which is responsible for the production of energy. My calculated guess was that I was experiencing mitochondrial dysfunction and thus required an energy boost. This peptide was miraculous in repairing my energy when I had none and helped me immensely in terms of having the stamina to get back my physical strength.

INFLAMMATORY DAMAGE

TB 500 and BPC 157: A combination of both peptides reduced inflammation throughout my body, and because I experienced severe body aches, joint aches, and a lot of inflammation, I concluded it was fibromyalgia.

TB-500 is an amino acid peptide sequence shown to improve blood vessel growth, regulate wound healing, decrease inflammation, and reduce oxidative damage in the heart and central nervous system. Additionally, it's known to regenerate and remodel injury to damaged tissue.

The sister product, BPC-157, is a peptide body protection compound known to exhibit analgesic characteristics that significantly accelerate collagen formation. The foundation of BPC-157 comes from protein that already exists within the stomach, and can accelerate healing processes throughout the body. I used a combination of BPC-157 and TB-500 daily.

IMMUNE SYSTEM

Thymosin Alpha 1: Thymosin Alpha 1 is a naturally occurring peptide from the thymus gland, between the chest and the lungs. It has been known to restore and enhance immune function, and has been used in the past as a treatment for immunocompromised patients. There is also preliminary data that suggests Thymosin Alpha 1 enhances vaccine response, making the latest vaccines function better within the body and fight infection more potently. It has abundant antiviral properties and is currently on the way to being a popular and accepted treatment for respiratory ailments like long Covid.

Thymalin: This is a synthetic peptide that I have prescribed in cytolytic consultations, but has recently been known to bring forth immune system support. It works by tracking down cell imbalances in your body and altering natural killer (NK) cell activity. It is also being researched now as a kind of peptide that can increase vaccine protection, similar to Thymosin Alpha 1.

REBUILDING MUSCLE MASS

GHRP-2 and GHRP-6: These products are growth hormone–releasing peptides critical because of tremendous tissue wasting and loss of muscle. GHRP-2 is referred to as a growth hormone–releasing peptide and has been shown to improve muscle growth, regulate the immune system, and improve sleep cycles. I used it every day and it also helped significantly with my appetite. GHRP-6 is effective in building healthy tissue. It exerts positive effects on the heart muscle and memory formation by protecting brain tissue, much of which I felt had been damaged as a consequence of Covid.

ANTI-AGING

Epitalon: This peptide works as an agent to fight aging and helps with age reversal—and Covid *definitely* accelerated my own aging process. When I was released from the hospital, I had aged forty years in twenty days. I did not recognize myself when I looked in the mirror. My friends and clients said I went from looking vital, a few decades younger than I actually was, to looking ancient— twenty or thirty years *older* than I actually was. Epitalon was essential to reversing the havoc that my hospital stay wreaked. It is a potential modulator of telomerase—a naturally occurring enzyme that maintains telomeres—the essential part of human cells that affects how our cells age and prevents them from shortening during cell division.

BRAIN BOOSTERS

PRL-8-53: Despite its clunky name, PRL-8-53 is actually a very simple and powerful peptide, sometimes categorized as a nootropic, that greatly improves memory, information retention, and general cognition. The supplement is made from components of benzoic acid, a natural compound found in several household foods, like berries and dairy products. PRL-8-53 improved my cognition not only at the level at which I functioned thirty to forty years ago, but also improved mental stimulation that I had lost with long Covid. I also found that it affected my mood and sentence construction.

Piracetam: I call this particular product the "granddaddy of all." I found it especially helpful in waking me up and enabling me to be much more alert so I could focus and pay attention with greater immediacy. Piracetam specifically can help with stiffened cell membranes, allowing your brain and blood vessels to function correctly. Piracetam is specifically helpful in aiding memory and brain function, which can be beneficial while abstaining from coffee or caffeinated drinks during recovery.

Coluracetam: Considered a cognitive-enhancing supplement that acts as a mood enhancer with particular effect on relieving depression. It is a member of the racetam family, which means it comes directly from the original, piracetam.

Qualia (Qualia Mind): This particular dietary supplement is one I consider a fabulous catchall. I am outlining a specific section for it, as opposed to my typical ingredient-based approach, because of its multi-hyphenate nature, hybrid build, and effectiveness. I take Qualia Mind every day and know I'm getting something of everything to make my brain perform better. It includes a variety of nootropic substances as well as natural, vitamin-based supplements, which combine to make a potent and radically integral solution. This particular product could also be utilized in the Motivation and Mood Enhancing section below.

Noopept: A cognitive-enhancing supplement that improves focus, memory, and attention. It has a similar effect to piracetam, but it has a smaller dosage recommendation.

MOTIVATION AND MOOD ENHANCING

Bromantane: Instead of coffee, I find this supplement a profound motivational tool. This particular nootropic greatly improves brain function. My plan is to use a cap full of bromantane for two or three days, then take a break and start again two or three days later. I find it is very helpful for the first few days but then goes flat, so I have found it is best to self-administer in short spurts.

Aniracetam: This nootropic boosts memory, cognition, motivation, and also improves my mood tremendously.

Acetyl-L Carnitine: A nootropic critical for memory, cognitive skills, energy, and is used to reduce low affect or depression.

Alpha GPC: A brain motivator that aids in focus, learning, memory, and pushes the brain's dopamine level to lift the mood.

STRESS AND SLEEP HELPERS

Ashwagandha: This is a powerful herb, a plant-based product, with multiple benefits for sleep, as well as reduction of stress, anxiety, and depression. Ashwagandha is often referred to as providing an "instant zen."

Bacopa Monnieri: An herb from traditional ayurvedic medicine, bacopa improves cognitive function, while potentially reducing depression and anxiety as well. It is a perennial plant that can improve sleep as well as reduce the effects of cortisol on your body. It can act as a profound stress regulator and helps with better brain function and memory improvement. Bacopa is a plant-based product, as well.

Phosphatidylserine: This supplement is a fatty nutrient that both covers and protects the cells in your brain and carries messages between them, enabling your mind and memory to be sharp. Known to improve thinking skills and age-related decline in mental and cognitive function, additional benefits include help with sleep and a reduction of stress.

GENERAL SLEEP PRODUCTS

This is a comprehensive list of the remaining products that I use. I encourage you to take the smallest doses and see how they work, either alone or together. I may use all of them at night, and sometimes more than I have listed here. But it is most important at early stages to experiment with singular doses and track their effects. The products I use are:

- *L-Serine*
- *L-Glycine*
- *Melatonin*
- *P-5-P*
- *GABA*
- *Decaffeinated Green Tea Extract*
- *CBD*
- *5HTP*
- *Magnolia Extract*
- *Qualia Sleep*

NUTRACEUTICALS

Nutraceuticals are the umbrella term that includes vitamins, amino acids, antioxidants, minerals, various plant-based herbal products, mushrooms, and cannabis. Because of the vague grouping of nutraceuticals at large, each section will contain its own description for proper, specific categorization. Please note that I only include product recommendations for some of these supplements. The products I do recommend are from sources with which I trust and have an extensive rapport. Otherwise, I recommend acquiring the highest quality product at your own discretion.

AMINO ACIDS

Amino acids are molecules that combine to form proteins and together are the building blocks of life itself. While the body needs approximately twenty different amino acids to grow and function properly, only nine are essential—among those you may recognize are leucine, lysine, tryptophan, and valine. The best sources of essential amino acids are animal proteins like meat, eggs, and poultry. The ones I suggest increase vasodilation, circulation, and regulate blood pressure.

Agmatine: Agmatine is a chemical product found in plants and other natural sources, made from an amino acid called arginine. It can improve conditions involved in brain function, as well as improving chronic nerve pain and athletic performance. It can also aid in general endurance and provide a boost in workouts or at a low point of mood or motivation. The product I recommend is **Agmatine** from **Nootropic Depot**.

L-arginine and L-citrulline: I find that these two amino acids work best in tandem, as both combine to create nitric oxide in the body, an important signal-caller that can improve cellular responsiveness. Nitric oxide also improves immune and nervous system function at a high level. It also expands and dilates both blood and oxygen flow to various parts of the body, an essential function. This improves muscle strength, endurance, cardiac health, and lowers blood pressure. Because of the improvement to circulation, it can benefit neuropathy in hands and feet, both of which I experienced in my hospital stay. This process additionally maximizes your circulatory system. The product I recommend is **AngiNOX** from **Xymogen**. Another product that can provide the same function of arginine and citrulline is **Vasophil Sachets** from **Integrative Therapeutics**.

ANTIOXIDANTS

Antioxidants are substances that inhibit the "rusting" of your body. In medical terms, this process is known as oxidation and is the result of burnout from aging or illness. The Harvard School of Medicine says there are hundreds, if not thousands, of antioxidants, but these are the ones I use in my early morning glass of water, beverage, or smoothie since they perform multiple functions. **Important:** Do not forget that you need fruits and vegetables for antioxidant support as well.

Glutathione: I call this product the king of all antioxidants, and it is superb for promoting tissue building, anti-aging liver function, heart health, as well as improving pulmonary function. To be specific, glutathione acts as an important antioxidant fighting free radicals—those molecules that can damage your body's cells. Glutathione decreases as you get older, which plays into poor health, so it plays a larger role after great illness or at a later stage of life. Glutathione supplements provide intracellular support and promote healthy cell function and healthy aging, detoxification, a healthy immune response, amino acid transport across cell membranes, and enhance the antioxidant activity of vitamins C and E. The product I recommend is **S-acetyl Glutathione** from **Xymogen**.

N-Acetyl-L-Cysteine (NAC): As I have mentioned before, this antioxidant supports pulmonary function and overall wellness, including the liver and kidneys. NAC supports overall respiratory function, glutathione production, and detoxification. The benefits include promoting lung tissue and respiratory function, support of cellular antioxidant defense systems, and tissue detoxification. It also improves brain health and acts against inflammation, by loosening mucus in air passages, helping the bronchial tubes. I relied on NAC to build back my lung functions. The product I recommend is **N-Acetyl-L-Cysteine** from **Pure Encapsulations**.

Alpha Lipoic Acid: This antioxidant may reduce inflammation and skin aging, promote healthy nerve function, and lower heart disease risk.

Nicotinamide Adenine Dinucleotide (NAD): Works in the body as a little steam engine to kick-start your "cellular engines" or mitochondria and create energy.

Astaxanthin: This powerful antioxidant is hugely helpful for vision, and since my vision has been particularly affected, I take a handful a day. It is also great for your heart health. It is a carotenoid, providing a multitude of health benefits, including anti-inflammatory and immune-enhancing properties and DNA repair.

Resveratrol: A potent antioxidant helper to lower blood pressure and boost the immune system. Most people are familiar with the benefits of red wine on the cardiovascular system and with anti-aging because red wine contains the powerful compound resveratrol, which also promotes healthy platelet function.

MSM: A substance helpful with joint inflammation and relief of muscle stiffness. It is a natural sulfur-containing compound found in plants, animals, and humans and helps promote a healthy immune system along with improving healthy hair, skin, and nails.

Pycnogenol: An extract of French pine bark that improves muscle energy and boosts nitric oxide levels; it has widely been used to improve circulation, high blood pressure, and overall cardiovascular health.

MINERALS

Minerals are one of the two most used supplements by American adults, along with general vitamins. Minerals are a blanket term for several of the components that are frequently included in popular dietary supplements, foods, and beverages. The minerals I find the most use out of are in the zinc and magnesium families, though there is also added benefit in calcium, selenium, and more, which can be provided through the functional food habits I have recommended. Magnesium, specifically, offers help in these different forms for sleep, stress reduction, and improving bowel movement.

Magnesium Threonate: This supplement is a powerful agent of change, and it is especially popular among other magnesium products because of its wide-reaching effects, specifically that it can raise magnesium levels within the brain. Though it is uncommon for people with a strong, healthy diet to require extra magnesium, after an illness or with an unhealthy diet, a magnesium deficiency can be extremely costly. Threonate can promote cognitive health and provide an avenue for magnesium to easily reach the brain. Magnesium levels are essential within the brain and nervous system to avoid potential brain-related illness.

Magnesium Taurate: This is a hybrid form of magnesium that also contains the amino acid taurine. In tandem, this combination can help regulate blood sugar in the body. It was certainly helpful in managing my high blood pressure after the hospital and to keep it low as I was eating a lot and gaining mass.

Magnesium Glycinate: Due to its multi-hyphenate reach within the body, magnesium can play a role in a plethora of the body's functions, including sleep. I use magnesium glycinate as one of my sleep aids primarily, and it can also greatly help with bowel function. It is a very calming supplement with widespread use.

Krebs Zinc: This supplement provides a combination of five forms of zinc critical for rebuilding energy. This particular formula helps the body absorb zinc more easily and is important for wound healing as well as regaining a sense of taste and smell. These five unique nutrients allow for optimum cycling of cells to boost energy and more. It is additionally key for tissue repair and integrity, immunity, and antioxidant protection.

ESSENTIAL OILS

Essential oils are compounds that often include extracts from plants and other organisms. They are known to have anti-inflammatory, immunomodulatory, bronchodilatory, and antiviral properties, and I use many of the ones listed below.

Fish Oil: This is the most popular and well-known type of essential oil used today. It is known most frequently as a provider of omega-3. But specifically, the two most important types of omega-3s that fish oil provides are eicosapentaenoic acid (EPA) and docosahexaenoic acid (DHA). These fatty acids can reduce heart disease, provide pain relief, boost muscle strength, and improve physical performance. Beyond just standard fish oil, I also recommend both krill and cod liver oil within the umbrella.

Flaxseed Oil: This is another popular type of essential oil that is high in a different omega-3 called alpha-linolenic acid (ALA). This fatty acid can decrease inflammation and swelling, which makes it optimal for those with arthritis or arthritic conditions. It can also be used for regression of blood pressure levels and preventing heart disease.

Medium-Chain Triglycerides: Also known as MCT oil, this supplement is used in tandem with its counterpart, long-chain triglycerides, which are more common in foods. Both have health benefits, but medium-chain fats are easier to digest, making their impact more quickly felt. The MCT oil that I use comes from palm kernel oil, but can also be derived from coconut oil. As I said, it can be used to help digest fats as well as providing energy and reducing inflammation.

Sesame Seed Oil: This essential oil is completely separate from the sesame oil used in cooking. Sesame seed oil has potential health benefits that can aid in wear and tear due to aging and help prevent cardiovascular disease. There is also preliminary evidence that it can reduce inflammation, as well.

Olive Oil: I have mentioned how olive oil is essential to use while cooking for both weight gain and muscle retention, but it also has health benefits beyond nutritional value. Olive oil has plenty of fatty acids and vitamin E. It is easily absorbable and contains several other key vitamins and nutrients.

Coconut Oil: This is another oil often used in cooking, but I use it as a carrier oil for several uses, including promoting hair and skin health. It is rich in antioxidants and I like its nourishing qualities, as well.

Black Seed Oil Very high in antioxidants, black seed oil may be beneficial for treating various skin conditions and lowering blood sugar and cholesterol. It is a plant-based nutrient that can reduce inflammation and relax muscles in the airway, which helps with asthma, asmatic symptoms, and respiratory issues. It is clearly applicable to improving lung function. The product I recommend is **Black Seed Oil** from **Triquetra Health**.

Dandelion Oil: This oil is believed to help detox the liver and calm the stomach and nervous system. Like many other essential oils, it also has anti-inflammatory qualities. The product I recommend is **Dandelion Root** from **Nature's Way**.

Oregano Oil: This oil has a history of use for immune support dating back to ancient Greece and Rome and is popular today for the same reason. It is a prevalent and powerful antioxidant. The product I recommend is **Oregano Oil Immune Support** from **Nature's Way**.

PLANT OR HERBAL-BASED PRODUCTS

The following products are solely made from plants and herbs and can maintain health with natural healing properties. Many popular prescription drugs, as well as some of the supplements I have mentioned before, are made from plant products, but these are strictly plant-based and regulated by the FDA as pure. Some of them are entire plants themselves and others are whittled down to their most essential elements.

Tudca: This is a supplement that can help with liver damage and stimulate bile flow. Tudca may also support the gallbladder, digestive system, kidneys, eyes, and brain. It contains elements to tackle multiple cognitive problems. It detoxifies, improves digestion, and regulates blood sugar. It may play a role in blocking respiratory infections throughout the body.

Quercetin: This is a critical antioxidant and anti-inflammatory supplement with properties that may aid in the prevention of neurodegenerative diseases.

Medical Cannabis: I found medical cannabis a lifesaver for my state of mind, and either as an edible or smoked, it raised my mood and continues to be critical for my state of mind and sleep.

Rutin: Citrus-flavored rutin, which supports blood circulation and a healthy heart, is an antioxidant useful in treating osteoarthritis and inflammatory conditions.

Curcumin: Produced by plants and sold as an herbal supplement, curcumin is used for the treatment of chronic diseases, inflammatory bowel disease, pancreatitis, and arthritis, among other conditions.

Sceletium Tortuosum: A plant-based supplement to reduce anxiety, enhance mood, and promote relaxation.

Ergothioneine: A mushroom extract and amino acid that can be used for liver damage, diabetes, heart disease, and cataracts.

VITAMINS

We have come a very long way since vitamin C became a staple in our households, but there is a full alphabet of others we need. Vitamins are nutrients the body needs to function and fight off disease. Our bodies use vitamins to develop and function normally, but since the body can't produce them, think of A, C, D, E, K, choline, and the various BS as your friends. Always eat foods high in these vitamins.

6

My Long Covid Personal Program for Rebuilding My Body and Immune System

Understanding how various supplements work in the body allows you to see their value. Incorporating nutraceuticals and other supplements into our bodies is about strengthening ourselves now for what may be ahead. It is essential to make our future selves grateful for our own foresight.

I formulated and laid out this specific course of supplements and nutraceuticals that I used to target my compromised immune system, exhaustion, mental apathy, traumatized state of mind, and wasted body. Most people who have gotten Covid or even suffer from long Covid, in my experience, will not need to focus on every single one of these issues. What I experienced was uniquely damaging. I had to become my own guide, cheerleader, and the champion of gaining back my health and stability. I had no guidelines, no map, no blueprint, no assistance or intelligence coming in from the medical community, nothing at all. I was my own light and I had to figure out what to do, and I had to do it quickly.

What follows is the exact combination that I used personally, but I recommend all of the supplements I have already mentioned. It is tailored to my specific needs and recovery. This is more of a complete list of my recovery setup. Some of these I have defined before, but many of them are additional ones that I have used and still use.

I need to remind you that these are based on my own personal use and experience. If you choose to take these products, follow the directions as put forth by your general practitioner and see how your body responds. I always recommend being cautious at first no matter what. This is my personal program and what I follow.

MY PERSONAL PROGRAM LIST FOR RECOVERING FROM LONG COVID

PHOSPHATIDYLSERINE

BACOPA

NAC

GLUTATHIONE

ASTAXANTHIN

KREBS ZINC

FISH OIL

BLACK SEED OIL

TUDCA

ERGOTHIONEINE

MULLEIN LEAF: Reduces inflammatory lung conditions, often used in a variety of issues from bronchitis to cough and congestion.

PLANTAIN: Extremely useful as it soothes, softens, and hydrates the respiratory system due to its high mucilage content.

NMN: An energy-enhancing nutrient that improves cellular and mitochondrial function and prevents age-related changes in gene expression. A relative of both niacin and vitamin B3.

PQQ: A longevity nutrient that raises blood flow to the cerebral cortex aiding attention, thinking, and memory. Improves sleep and mood. It protects nerve cells against damage while also supporting energy and mitochondrial function. May reduce inflammation in the brain.

ACETYL-L-CARNITINE ARGINATE: This is a carnitine derivative that promotes youthful cellular energy metabolism along with mood and nervous system competence. It is a powerful antioxidant that also encourages cognitive function.

BUTYREX: A nutrient compound that provides colon cells with energy, reduces inflammation, and reduces risk of diseases like Crohn's, irritable bowel syndrome, and leaky gut syndrome.

REPHYLL: Has potent anti-inflammatory, antimicrobial, antibacterial, and antioxidant properties. It also relieves anxiety and chronic pain. It may specifically improve joint problems along with pain management. It is a unique extract of black pepper clove, rosemary, and more.

ZEMBRIN: This plant-based nutrient elevates mood, has a calming, anti-stress effect, and improves serenity, motivation, and energy.

NATTOKINASE: Natto comes from fermented soy beans. It is shown to dissolve blood clots, maintain blood vessel structure, and lower blood pressure.

NADH: This vitamin-like compound can reduce fatigue and increase energy, and mental and sports performance. In combination with CoQ10, it can alleviate chronic fatigue.

FRENCH MARITIME PINE BARK EXTRACT: This is a potent antioxidant that supports blood flow and reduces inflammation, while improving both brain function and immunity. It likely improves muscle performance during exercise.

VITAMIN C: Ascorbic acid, critical for the growth, development, and formation and repair of all body tissues, from the formation of collagen to proper immune function and the maintenance of cartilage, bones, and teeth.

VITAMIN D: Among the multiple benefits of this powerhouse vitamin are supporting immune brain and nervous system health, supporting lung and heart function, and influencing the genes involved in cancer development.

PROPIONYL-L-CARNITINE: This nutrient plays a role in increasing ATP generation; hence it is key in energy production. It is also a potent antiradical agent and likely protects tissues from severe oxidative damage. It spans the therapeutic spectrum of protecting against cardiovascular diseases.

BRANCHED-CHAIN AMINO ACIDS (ESPECIALLY LEU-CINE): This family of amino acids builds muscle, decreases muscle fatigue, slows muscle loss, and alleviates muscle soreness. Leucine, in particular, aids in the natural production of growth hormone, and additionally, further supports muscle growth. It activates mTor in your tissues, further regulating the production of new tissue, especially muscle.

THEANINE: An extract of tea that promotes sleep and relaxation by multiple contributions to brain performance. Key among them is increased levels of GABA in the brain, as well as lowering excitatory chemicals that contribute to stress and anxiety. It has also been associated with positive mood enhancement.

BOSWELLIA: A key anti-inflammatory that can aid with body aches and pains, arthritis, and joint and muscle pains.

CORYDALIS: A plant extract that improves sleep, reduces insomnia, and is effective in reducing inflammatory pain. It can also be used for mild depression, nerve damage, and tremors.

EMOXYPINE: This nutrient exercises anxiolytic, anti-stress, and anticonvulsant actions, while improving cerebral circulation. It also promotes both cardioprotective and anti-atherosclerotic function.

ARTEMISININ: A plant-based product that has been used to combat malaria. It is also a hedge against pancreatitis (which I developed from Covid), and it normalized both my lipase and amylase levels. It also exhibits cell repair, and immune enhancing properties.

GLYCINE: An amino acid that spans across the regulation of the immune system, from limiting inflammation to improving pain perception, sleep, and mood.

MAGNESIUM TAURINE: An amino acid required for aspects of brain formation, long-term memory formation, and improved sleep.

MUCUNA: A tropical plant that boosts depleted dopamine levels, alleviating depression and improving sleep. It is an antioxidant booster. It also may fight pathogens, inflammation, and have a normalizing effect on blood pressure and male reproductive function.

5 HTP: This nutrient helps raise serotonin, regulating mood and behavior, exerting a positive effect on sleep, mood, anxiety, appetite, and pain sensation.

HYPOXEN: A nutrient that improves oxygen utilization, by increasing tissue respiration in the brain, liver, and heart muscle. It does so under extreme conditions that are accompanied by a lack of oxygen.

L-THREONINE: An essential amino acid also used to aid a variety of autoimmune disorders, to reduce anxiety and improve sleep. It also aids muscles and connective tissue to maintain elasticity. It is an essential part of magnesium theanine, as well.

BIOFLAVONOIDS: Bioflavonoids are a large family of fruit-based pigments with potent antioxidant and anti-inflammatory properties, which reduce chronic pain, improve cardiovascular circulation, and helping to prevent neurodegenerative diseases.

L-SERINE: An amino acid that improves sleep initiation and reduces nighttime awakening; it also improves memory and thinking skills while reducing long-term neurological damage.

ANCESTRAL SUPPLEMENTS: A comprehensive line of desiccated organs from organic grass-fed beef out of New Zealand. Everything from bone marrow extract to spleen, beef pancreas, heart, and brain. I developed severe anemia and low/small red blood cells, and a combination of these extracts rapidly corrected this condition along with providing energy improvements.

SPERMIDINE: Critical extract in that it may play a role in inhibiting multiple hallmarks of aging along with improving vaccine protection. Its effects mimic those of calorie restriction, thus providing an additional hack in keeping cells healthier and younger.

AC-11: An extract of cat's-claw, which boosts cells repair mechanisms, DNA regeneration, and immune support. It supports apoptosis, which is our body's ability to clear out damaged cells.

BETAINE ANHYDROUS: This product helps with metabolizing homocysteine, which is involved in several functions of the brain, blood, heart, and more. Buildup of homocysteine can slow blood flow and hinder neural function.

CALCIUM ALPHA KETOGLUTARATE: I use this in powder form as it plays a critical role in fighting premature aging and extending health span through a multitude of pathways. It is an up-and-coming cinolytic product that will be top of the line soon.

ANTIHISTAMINES: Remarkably, this over-the-counter medicine for allergic reactions has had a drastic reinvention in recent months. Preliminary studies showed that antihistamines can help curb long Covid symptoms, and I found them very effective, specifically non-drowsy medication.

The following are products I find effective and recommend:

Wholly Immune from **Allergy Research Group**

This product offers total immune and nutrient support. It is a comprehensive powdered blend of nutrients and herbs designed to support general nutrition, immune system function, liver detoxification, and provide antioxidant support. Included are vitamins B2, B6, B12, and folate in bioactive coenzyme forms.

Buffered Ascorbic Acid Capsules from **Pure Encapsulations**

This particular vitamin C supplement is for sensitive individuals and the dosage is one capsule between one and four times daily with or between meals.

SelenoExcell from **Natural Factors**

A selenium complex produced by yeast—and Maitake 404 blend—a proprietary blend of whole mushroom mycelium powers.

Neuro Shroom Extract Powder from **PrimalHerb**

Medicinal mushrooms have documented effects against infections and inflammatory disorders and may be helpful in the treatment of the severe lung inflammation that often follows Covid-19 infection.

Quercetin from **Pure Encapsulations**

A dietary supplement belonging to a class of water-soluble plant pigments called bioflavonoids that cannot be produced in the human body. Quercetin promotes cardiovascular health, helps to boost immunity, fights inflammation, combats allergies, and helps exercise performance.

Vitamin D3 from **Pure Encapsulations**

Vitamin D3 enhances calcium absorption and retention, which is key in supporting healthy bones and may play a role in cardiovascular, colon, and cellular health. Because vitamin D levels tend to decline with age, decreased exposure to sunlight, a vegetarian diet, or low intake of Vitamin D–fortified foods, this is a key vitamin.

Melatonin from **Pure Encapsulations**

Melatonin is a hormone produced by the pineal gland, the organ that regulates the body's wake/sleep/wake cycle. Melatonin nutritionally augments the body's natural sleep cycle.

Nattosyn from **Douglas Laboratories**

A combination of nattokinase, hesperidin methyl chalcone, and pomegranate extract, this is designed to provide comprehensive support for circulatory health. Traditionally,

Asian cultures have incorporated significant amounts of soy products in their diets, and one such product, natto, is a type of vegetable cheese produced from the fermentation of soy with a non-pathogenic bacterium, Bacillus natto.

Thymulus from Nature's Way

Your immune health is connected to the well-being of the thymus gland. Thymus extract may help to combat respiratory infections and asthma attacks triggered by an overactive immune system. Thymus extract is also used to treat viral infections due to its immune-boosting properties. It is also an alternative therapy for autoimmune diseases, which may flare during an immune assault from Covid-19.

IgG 2000 CWP from Xymogen

Supports immune function by providing immunoglobulins and supports the body's normal gut repair pathways.

Super Omega 3 from Life Extensions

Helps support cardiovascular, cognitive, and eye health with a concentrated and purified source of omega-3 fatty acids.

Theracurmin HP from Integrative Therapeutics

Reduces inflammation, pain, and improves immune system function.

Luteolin Powder from ePothex

Luteolin is found in many herbs, fruits, and vegetables and has its medicinal origins in Chinese medicine. Contemporary studies have indicated that it could inhibit viral infection symptoms in long Covid patients.

MY SMOOTHIE

My morning smoothie is one of the most important aspects to my daily life. Since I returned home from the hospital, and could stand up on two feet, I have been preparing this smoothie for myself, mixing and matching certain ingredients to fully optimize what it can do for me. Before my smoothie, though, in order to maintain a good bowel movement and to offset the constipation that may occur with the paleo diet, I used flax and chia seed powder and inulin powder first thing in the morning in a big glass of water. I did this every morning to reduce inflammation in my bowel and increase its capacity for probiotics to adhere to the bowel wall. This is usually now followed by a smoothie.

In other words, since probiotics, a key component for managing both the general health of the immune system and improving cognitive function, need a sticky surface to latch onto in the bowel wall, the prebiotics were the first thing I would consume on an empty stomach. Just in case you may have forgotten, the bowel is approximately thirty feet long. That is an extreme amount of surface to cover, and the importance of bowel health became critically important to me. I began immediately by replacing my probiotics as soon as possible once I returned home. After the massive amount of medications, antibiotics, and poor quality food I consumed in the hospital, every aspect of my diet, and my supplements, became critical to rebuilding my body and, at the very least, start rebuilding my bowel flora, my microbiome.

To this day, I continue to follow the same regimen despite modifying my initial diet. After the prebiotics, and the smoothie itself, I begin with my first handful of multiple supplements and nutraceuticals that, by category, increase my mental clarity and energy levels while reducing inflammation and increasing my energy. The ingredients and recipes for the smoothies are listed below. I have described many of these products in the previous chapter.

I then prepare my morning smoothie, which includes all the nutrients needed to nourish me properly and wake me up. I include some probiotics and an amino acid mix, made of L-arginine, citrulline, and agmatine or Vasophil Sachets to boost my nitric oxide levels. Included as well is additional citrulline, an amino acid made from both watermelon and beetroot powder, high in nitrous oxide, as well the amino acid beta-alanine, which increases the production of L-carnosine to reduce exhaustion, improve endurance, and lessen muscle fatigue. I add in green tea extract for a bit of caffeine as well as flax or chia powder, with organic blueberries. There is a bevy of supplements that I have included that also build muscle mass, strengthen my heart, increase circulation within muscles, help my mental alertness, and alleviate pain. Here is the recipe:

- 1–2 container scoops Mixed Beverage Base
  This represents the base for any and all my
  smoothies. Look for products that are based

on pea and rice extracts. The ones I use are highly fortified to reduce inflammation, detox liver pathways, and provide a gentle and highly supportive food for the colon. The two products I recommend are **Ultraclear RENEW** from **Metagenics** and **OptiCleanse** from **Xymogen**.

- ½ tsp. Broccoli Sprout Powder
  Super rich in sulforaphane, this powder is an organic compound with neuroprotective, anti-inflammatory, anti-microbial, anti-cancer, anti-aging, and anti-diabetic properties. It also can protect against cardiovascular and neurodegenerative diseases.

- ½ tsp. Inulin Powder

- 1 tsp. Flaxseed Powder with or without Chia Seed Powder

- L-Arginine and Citrulline

- 1 tsp. Green Powder
  A key part of the smoothie, green powder is a dietary supplement that can help mineral and vitamin intake, and has immune system support built in. The product I recommend is **Green Protein Alchemy** from **HealthForce**

SuperFoods, which has everything from spirulina to barley grass sprouts.

- ⅔ tsp. Calcium Alpha Ketoglutarate

- Probiotics
  An example combination would be ¼ tsp. each Natren Probiotics Acidophilus, Bifido, Bulgaricum, Lactobacillus Rhamnounosus, 1–2 capsules Solace, 1 capsule Target-X, 1-2L Plantarum Kaged Muscle, Primal Defense

- 1 tsp. AMLA or Gooseberry Powder
  Besides its richness in vitamin C and fiber, gooseberry powder also aids in the protection of the pancreas and the immune system. Additionally, it can protect against a slew of chronic conditions.

- 1 Container **Scoop Collagen Peptides** from **Ancient Nutrition**
  For repair of damaged skin, improving skin elasticity, and reducing skin dryness. Peptides here also improve damaged hair and nails. After leaving the hospital, I was all hanging skin and my hair was falling out. I find this critical to rebuilding healthy skin.

- Almond Milk / Coconut Milk to desired consistency/dilution

- Handful of Frozen Mixed Berries

- ½ Avocado (optional)

ALL PRODUCTS ARE ADDED TO BLENDER. MIX TO DESIRED CONSISTENCY. FLAVORS CAN BE ADDED SUCH AS GROUND COCOA OR VANILLA.

7

Additional Therapies and Alternative Healing

There are a host of alternative and progressive treatments that are becoming more and more mainstream. In both my professional and general life, there is a growing awareness that there are ways to cope with various issues—aches, pains, recovery from injury—that exist beyond traditional medicine. These practices can also restore a sense of well-being, which I specifically needed after long Covid. All around New York City, in fact, there has been large swathes of IV drip therapy, mild hyperbaric oxygen therapy, and intramuscular shots (IM), as the prevalence and use of these practices becomes widely known and accepted as potentially beneficial. Before going through with any of these treatments, I just ask that you do your homework, make sure the places are legitimate, super clean, and follow Covid protocols. The main way this can backfire is if there is a Covid outbreak amidst the healing process. I have already discussed a few alternative healing methods previously that I will not include here, like intermittent fasting, ice baths, lung exercises, and medicinal cannabis, but they could also qualify in this section as well. Here are some of the therapies I use and recommend:

Acupuncture: A key ingredient in traditional Chinese medicine, acupuncture can be an extremely helpful remedy for pain treatment. It can stimulate nerves, muscles, and general tissue that may have been damaged. Preliminary studies have shown that acupuncture has improved Covid patients' inflammation and has regulated general nervous system function.

Vitamin IV Therapy: I have had several clients come into my office, asking about IV vitamin therapy, most of them having tried it before to cure a hangover or jet lag. And although it can be effective in these (usually cosmetic) cases, IV vitamin therapy can be used for more serious wellness and it can be utilized to great effect. An IV session, in essence, is a process through which one can receive a liquid mixture of vitamins and minerals directly into a vein, accelerating the process of ingestion of said products into the bloodstream. Going in for an IV session helped my immune system get back on track. It was incredibly helpful for me in particular because my weak stomach did not have the capacity for quick turnaround in feeling the effects of certain supplements, and the IV process greatly increased their effectiveness. IV vitamin therapy can be highly effective for people with illnesses that could interfere with nutrient absorption, like long Covid.

Bodywork: The majority of the bodywork I did in recovery came in the form of deep tissue massage. As I said in my "Routine" section, I would partake once a week or so, with very intense sessions focusing on reducing inflammation, and getting to the core of the problems I had with both my deep and soft tissue. The sessions can be painful at first, but the result is a great sense of flexibility in the midst of severe inflammation, as well as incredible sleep benefits.

Ozone Therapy: Also known as 10-Pass, ozone therapy is the safest, most efficient way to transport ozone to the body. Ozone has been shown to treat several of the issues I faced throughout long Covid, like inflammation, pneumonia, and some of my neurological conditions.

Ketamine: Yes, ketamine is absolutely a common recreational drug, but it has also been scientifically proven to aid in mitigating the severity of PTSD symptoms. I experienced rapid improvement with ketamine as an aid, and my neural response was robust after my sessions. It was more effective than any pharmaceutical I had tried previously to curb my traumatic responses and anxiety.

Although I alternate treatments depending on how I feel, the three consistent favorites that work for me are:

The Infrared Sauna: I used the infrared sauna primarily to accelerate healing and repair. Infrared is not always an accessible option, and I find that there are benefits to regular saunas as well, but with infrared, these benefits are increased tenfold. Infrared saunas differ from their normal counterparts by using light to create heat that warms the air, and the benefits are achieved at a lower temperature—I knew I might not have been able to handle the heat. The infrared sauna certainly aided in relaxation and general body therapy.

Cryotherapy: On the other side of the spectrum, I used cryotherapy, or "cold therapy," to reduce inflammation, swelling, and sore muscles. There have also been studies that have shown cryotherapy to boost immune health and strength. Additionally, cryo-chambers are made for one person at a time, so at the very least, there is very little potential for reinfection.

Hyperbaric Oxygen Therapy (HBO): I used HBO to increase oxygen into my tissue, reduce inflammation, and accelerate wound repair and healing. The process involves the inhalation of pure oxygen in pressurized settings, allowing the lungs to take in more oxygen than usual. That extra oxygen enters the bloodstream, providing aid when I was struggling with a suboptimal lung capacity.

DEVICES AND TOOLS

Sleep Devices

As I mentioned earlier, after my hospital stay, where I lingered in a twilight of bright lights and noise, never knowing what time it was and surrounded by gurneys ferrying dying patients in and out, I returned home unable to find sleep and capture the rest I desperately sought. No element is more crucial for recovery, and in fact, studies show one out of every three adults does not get enough sleep. I had to reach for any help, and so in addition to the products mentioned above, I learned about wearable sleep devices that can train the body to reach deep meditative sleep and reduce the anxiety that shows up in many, if not most, long Covid patients. Whichever of these devices you choose, understand that they are of fundamental help with general mood, well-being, and mental health.

Fitbit Alta 101: This product is a customizable fitness tracker. In addition to measuring your activity and exercise level, it can also continuously measure your sleep history, including hours slept and sleep patterns, as well as the hours of the day you were active or stationary. This particular model tracks the time you sleep and your movement during the night to help you understand sleep patterns. When I began to regulate my sleep after a period of great disturbance, I would check my Fitbit first thing in the morning to monitor my progress and gauge my sleep health in the process.

Oura Ring: The latest model of the Oura Ring monitors your heart rate around the clock, giving you the insights needed to make the most of your days and nights. The Oura Ring recognizes when your body and mind are relaxing, so you'll be up to date if you are taking enough breaks throughout the day and getting the recovery your body needs. Oura gets to know your unique, "normal" body temperature and picks up even the smallest changes with precise research-grade temperature sensors. My Oura Ring became crucial as I transitioned from being bedridden to working actively again. It helped me understand the waves of tiredness that I felt. I used it as my own personal "body boss," so I would not work myself to the point of endless fatigue.

Muse 2 and Muse 2 Plus: Brain Sensing Headband: This ingenious product has been referred to as a "digital sleeping pill." Muse 2 uses advanced EEG (electroencephalography) technology to respond to your mind, heart, and breath. Muse 2 is a comfy, brain-sensing headband that helps you understand and track how well you focus, sleep, and recharge so you can refocus during the day and recover each night. This device also includes excellent guided meditations!

NuCalm: NuCalm solves the riddle of safely and reliably managing stress and is the world's first and only patented neuroscience device clinically proven to reduce stress and improve sleep quality without drugs. NuCalm uses state-of-the-art applied neuropsychobiology and neuro bioinformatics to mimic the body's natural experience of a slowing brain and body function in preparation for sleep. A big selling point is that NuCalm guides your brain wave function to alpha and theta ranges and suspends you in parasympathetic nervous system dominance—a state of relaxation where you are physically incapable of experiencing stress.

Sana: Sana is a simple mask with headphones that carefully coordinates pulses of light and sound to guide the user into a deep state of relaxation, promoting increased recovery from fatigue.

Kokoon: What works to help you sleep and unwind is personal. There is no "one size fits all" solution when it comes to your relaxation. Kokoon works with you, your body, and your environment to create a personalized relaxation experience. The sleep-monitoring headphones pair with the MyKokoon app to monitor your sleep and give you personalized insights, improvements, and audio. I have used Kokoon every single night since I returned from the hospital, as it shuts out unnecessary noise and allows me peaceful sleep.

To Exercise the Mind and Body

HAELO PEMF Device: Referred to as a "next-gen device," PEMF uses a safe technology that emits sound frequencies to replenish cellular health. Elite athletes use it for relaxation and mood improvement, and it can provide the body with rhythmic symphonic frequencies to restore balance, boost immunity, and help with recovery and sleep. The HAELO PEMF has been referred to as a workout for your cells, which in turn helps optimize the whole body and its daily functions.

Hypervolt by Hyperice: The Hypervolt massage device features three speeds of rapid percussion that can be changed with a single button to cycle through whatever speed you need without interruption. Among other devices from Hyperice is the Normatec Leg Compression System that helps to improve circulation and oxygen distribution throughout the body.

Vielight: An amazing next-gen wearable headband, it is attached to a handheld device that enhances cerebral blood flow and brain metabolism. Mental acuity is enhanced by delivering light therapy to different points in the brain and can clear the brain fog many long Covid patients experience. Users claim the adjustable power is enormously helpful for those fighting acute anxiety.

Lung and Breathing Enhancers

Expand-A-Lung: A breathing resistance trainer, it is considered a breakthrough device for improving endurance through better breathing and lung function. Using this device significantly improves the strength of respiratory muscles and increases the volume of lung oxygen intake.

The Breather: This is the first drug-free device for those who suffer from shortness of breath and chronic illnesses resulting in respiratory weakness. It has been referred to as a home gym for your lungs.

The Airofit Pro: Based on smart technologies, the Airofit Pro measures your current lung function and personalizes a plan to improve your breathing; the improvement of lung capacity provides more energy and leads to significant well-being benefits. By strengthening your breathing muscles, you will not run out of breath doing everyday activities like climbing up stairs. I used it primarily to practice deep breathing exercises, as it tracked my lung capacity progress as I used it. When I began, I could only reach 1.4 (on a scale from 1 to 15). After four months, I reached a 10 on the scale.

O2: This device was my savior for quick oxygen intake after I returned from the hospital, as I vastly prefer it to the ventilators. Oxygen therapy was one of the practices that led me to get lung function back.

Mindfulness and Mindset

When you're in recovery from any catastrophic occurrence or illness, your mind also experiences trauma. It was hard for me to focus and quiet those anxious voices in my head that prevented me from resting. After an extended period in the hospital, as I have explained to friends and clients, I was absolutely exhausted and experienced a bit of a shock returning home, having been around so much death and nary an unmasked face for weeks and weeks. I often experienced triggers that led to my PTSD, and the apps I used were my primary path out of hell. Whatever it takes for you to become mindful and calm, do it!

These apps, along with my supplements, guided meditations, and books, allowed me to deal with my emotional collapse and I continue to use them every day. Key to recovery is understanding that the anxiety may reach a new level—that amygdala hijack, which can really happen at any time after a traumatizing experience. The result is anxiety and often paralyzing fear. The amygdala, housed within the temporal lobes, is responsible for processing fearful and threatening stimuli, especially fear and anxiety. It drives the fight or flee response. After Covid, I experienced an anxiety beyond anything I had suffered through before. These meditation apps are transformative and I was able to continue using them consistently. I cannot overstate their value in my recovery.

Waking Up: This guided meditation app created by Sam Harris should be used daily. It is not just another meditation app—*Waking Up* helps change the way you see the world. While the price may seem a bit steep, believe me, you need it—I certainly did. There are many courses with scientists, teachers, and scholars, enabling you to clear your mind and your negative thoughts, guiding you to experience loving-kindness. Begin with the course on fundamentals and learn the meditation practice. The purpose of meditation is to radically transform your sense of who you are and what you are. It can help you begin to understand your own mind and, eventually, experience enlightening changes due to these discoveries about yourself. By February 2022, just after a year after I had returned home from the hospital, I had 371 days in a row, 3,100 mindful minutes, and 516 sessions. It is life-changing.

Wim Hof App: Known as the god of ice water bathing and creator of his own breathing technologies, Wim Hof created the Wim Hof App to offer guided meditations and online courses, including a twenty-day cold shower challenge. Using this app has left me with a greater sense of clarity and higher amounts of dopamine in my system, so I automatically feel calmer. After religiously following this app, I can climb up five steps of stairs without effort, and I built up my lung capacity by being extremely vigorous with these exercises. I consider this app great for anxiety, while increasing circulation, energy, and power.

Calm and Headspace: These apps are two of the most popular guided meditation apps. Anything that helps with a good night's sleep and claims to make each day happier works for me

Tide: This app is a wonderful and extremely well-curated source of guided meditations, calming music, and nature sounds to bring the mind into stillness, sleep, and a quiet state.

Curable: This is an online program and app for those dealing with chronic pain. The app looks to help reduce the symptoms and calm the nervous system. For any doubters, Curable is compiled by a team of board-certified physicians, pain psychologists, and neuroscientists.

10% Happier: This is Dan Harris's terrific meditation app. His personal journey to finding meditation, and the book he wrote on the process, led Harris to create this meditation app, with coursework included.

Books

*Atomic Habits: An Easy & Proven Way to Build Good Habits & Break Bad On*es by **James Clear**: There is the most inspiring story behind this book, which kept me optimistic during my convalescence. *Atomic Habits* helped me see that just making 1 percent changes every day could amount to huge changes over time. Clear encourages tiny habit changes, which, just like atoms, have the ability to become mighty when repeated over and over again. This masterful book is a step-by-step system for creating good habits and breaking bad ones. Clear is not just a writer but a sought-after speaker at Fortune 500 companies and his backstory, which I mentioned in the introduction to this book, explains his expertise. I highly recommend this book.

Limitless: Upgrade Your Brain, Learn Anything Faster, and Unlock Your Exceptional Life by **Jim Kwik**: When Kwik was five, he suffered an accident that left him with brain damage and affected his ability to learn and function. He struggled greatly with memory retention and problem-solving skills during his childhood. Considered the world's premier brain coach, Kwik has written an owner's manual for mental expansion and brain fitness. By following his teachings, it taught me to reengage again and not just read but remember what I had read.

The Art of Impossible: A Peak Performance Primer by **Steven Kotler**: A *New York Times* best-selling author and executive director of the Flow Research Collective, Kotler is an expert on human performance. In *The Art of Impossible,* Kotler articulates what many peak performers intuitively know but can't explain, and breaks down the formula by giving readers the tools they need to accomplish their dreams.

Grit: The Power of Passion and Perseverance by **Angela Duckworth**: Duckworth is a pioneering psychologist pointing us toward the secret of outstanding achievement. It is not talent but, rather, a focused persistence called grit.

Boundless by **Ben Greenfield**: Greenfield is one of the premier authors in the field of health and fitness, and this book gives great insight into how Greenfield has managed to attain peak performance, and the tools that got him there.

Biohacker's Handbook: Upgrade Yourself and Unleash Your Inner Potential by **Jaakko Halmetoja**, **Olli Sovijärvi**, and **Teemu Arina**: This is a must-read if you are at all interested in the world of biohacking or body improvement. It gives a detailed analysis of how self-development and perfecting fundamentals can lead to the most optimal state of well-being.

Tribe of Mentors: Short Life Advice from the Best in the World by **Timothy Ferriss**: This is a completely unique book that features a compilation of outstanding advice from some of the thought leaders in the world whose advice I have sought out the most.

8

What About the Kids?

As my work and practice centers on anti-aging, I frequently work with clients who have children. My clients care about their families deeply—in fact, it is often a catalyst for my clients to pursue a healthier lifestyle, in order to spend more time with their children as well as maintain their health to extend further the time they may be able to spend with their families. Thus, children's health is also integral to my work in dealing with long Covid and the fallout of this illness, and we must not ignore children's well-being in this time of great peril, for you or potentially them. Your children take their guidance from you. Not only do they need proper diets and supplements, but they also need to follow your lead to further cultivate a sense of well-being throughout the family, from top to bottom. I want you to think about what messages parents and caregivers send when they provide mini plastic bags full of sweetened cereal bites, salty fish-shaped treats, and neon-orange doodles to toddlers sitting in strollers. Recently, a friend witnessed a very young child teething on a piece of pizza, and if you don't find that frightening, you're so wrong. In America, giving attention to children's health is often replaced with the easiest solution. While these treats and sweets can increase dopamine receptors in the short term, and may endear a child to their guardian, they have a profound impact on a child's development. There is so much more out there for parents and caretakers to provide for their children.

I understand how fortunate some of us are to have been exposed to the role lifestyle, fitness, and diet play in maintaining our well being. Whether your experience was like my own, and you found this path toward healthy living on your own, or it was passed down to you by a parent or relative, you must understand it is an absolute privilege. We are the entitled ones who can afford to provide ourselves with proper nutrition. But all parents need to be educated, because the dynamics within a family are passed on to our kids. If nutritional, smart living begins at a young age, it can engender a lifetime of well-being and robust health.

When we're talking about health, don't forget obesity in children has a direct effect on high blood pressure and diabetes, which then has a direct link to mortality. Obesity is the most prevalent bulwark toward healthy living in America today. If a child starts out overweight, the physical issues may, and usually will, only multiply. In the midst of a pandemic, obesity is number one in the list of conditions and can almost certainly compromise a young person's resistance and ability to securely handle viral infections, even with a relatively newer and unharmed immune system.

But cultivating this lifestyle is not a given—in fact, for many it can be quite difficult. I understand the schedules of working families and the rush to get kids off to school or handed off to caregivers. Childcare, in our current age of public health scarcity and ineffectuality, has become an increasingly difficult task. That being said, this sort of lifestyle can begin with small decisions. Meals and snacks can, cost-efficiently, become healthy ones. Fast-food choices, or quick options, do not have to be fried, highly processed, or lacking in vegetables and nutrients.

A few years ago, New York City–based pediatrician Natalie Geary and I co-wrote *Food Cure for Kids: A Nutritional Approach to Your Child's Wellness.* Geary, a Harvard graduate with a medical degree from Johns Hopkins Medical Center, who served on the faculty in Pediatrics at Columbia-Presbyterian Medical Center, Cornell-Weill Medical Center, Mount Sinai Medical Center, and NYU Medical Center, founded the vedaPURE company dedicated to infant and childhood nutrition, allergy, and wellness.

Geary and I teamed up over a mutual interest in nutrition and functional medicine, understanding the importance of food and supplements in treating illness and maintaining good health in children.

Now more than ever, we need to provide kids with their own defense systems and I'm sharing a small list of supplements you might add. But please keep in mind they are not a cure-all or substitute for a healthy diet. These supplements can only be properly utilized in addition to healthy living beyond functional medicine.

Remember, when a child eats a balanced diet, including a variety of fruits, vegetables, and proteins, they are quite literally feeding their own immune system, strengthening it as it ages. However, since many children go through phases where they don't eat as well as they probably should, the included supplements are specially recommended, as they are best designed for children's bodies. I have purposely not listed dosages because they differ according to your child's age and weight.

Be sure to read the manufacturer's label for dosage. Dosage depends on a child's weight, and not their age.

HEALTHY IMMUNE SYSTEM

Vitamins:

- **Kids Immune Gummy and Vitamin C, D, and Zinc Vegetarian Gummies** from **Garden of Life**
- **Vita-Kids Immune** from **Douglas Labs**

Multivitamins:

- **Metakids Multi Soft Chew** from **Metagenics**
- **Activnutrients Chew** from **Xymogen**

Vitamin D:

- **Metakids D3 Liquid** from **Metagenics**
- **Baby's Super Daily D3** from **Carlson Labs**

9

My So-Called Happy Ending

As Buddha might have said, "The problem is you think you have time."

I certainly thought I had time. In fact, I had lost sight of time. I did not even realize time had been passing. I bought into the illusion that I was going to be around for a while, even as I reached my seventies in that hospital bed. Now, one year later, I could not begin to explain where my seventieth year went.

Covid, and my long Covid complications, gave me a sense of uncertainty, one that I had been ignoring out of naivete.

In truth, I thought I was immortal.

I was the author of books on nutrition, age reversal, and optimum health and performance, with a client list who counted on me. Everything I did to stay super fit and be a motivator for my clients validated my way of life, my practice, and what I knew about staying young. But I almost lost all of it, in an instant. I almost lost it for good.

Covid almost killed me. I owned my hubris, and vanity was the least of my worries. Losing hope was the worst.

I think about death every day now, not fatalistically, but as a real entity, something that exists and happens to everyone. I'm very conscious that my battery pack will not last forever. I saw enough of the end to know that it is real. Even with my anti-aging practice and experience, I know I cannot actually deny the fact that, soon enough, I will be eighty years old.

And in what condition will I be? Throughout long Covid, I had chronic and severe joint pain, my muscles were completely shot, my vision was not working as it had been, and I was losing my hair in handfuls. With time and discipline, and the use of my protocols, I have begun to see my muscles return, my weight jump back up to a healthy amount, and my brain—which is my primary asset—has become sharper, and I can say that I have made as close to a full physical recovery as possible.

I can also report my energy and stamina have been revitalized in a big way. My vision has continued to improve. I feel sure that I owe this vast improvement to the use of my protocols, practices, and guidelines along with great determination and high discipline.

All I can say is that I am my own success story and experiment, and I have shown the ways in which my experiment has worked. This is not about how I saved my life, and I cannot guarantee to save yours. Despite my physical progress, I am not completely out of the woods. I don't know how anyone could claim to be, or how anyone could know. But what I do know is that I have maintained a critical level of discipline in following my protocols, even to this day.

I have, however, become especially aware that time now moves in an accelerated manner and that I may not meet all my goals. Though with this awareness, I've become more introspective. I'm more thoughtful in my actions, and I've developed patience that I never had. I fully needed to draw on patience after being locked in a hospital for three weeks, never knowing when I would be getting out or if I would even get out alive.

Before my Covid journey, I would put immense pressure on myself to achieve certain things right away. These days I recognize that everything is going to take time. In all earnestness, I have found what matters to me. In the past, I would wake up on the weekend and look to meet people, go to brunch, network, and be outside of myself. Today, my weekends are about gratitude. I follow my protocols in the morning and finish them off with my gratitude meditation. Now, the big event of my weekend is taking a walk in the park with my dog, then going home to read and write. I cannot believe how satisfying such a life has been for me.

I never had the inclination to value my solitude, my own space. I can now see, vividly, how I was afraid to be alone in the past. I had to fill up every moment with excitement, meeting people, attending events. Now, with my current mindset, that lifestyle is completely foreign to me. I have since lost my taste for it. Given the immense turnaround of my long Covid recovery, I cannot comprehend how much effort would be required to live that way—or even how I managed to do so. But feeling the way I do is not universal. How I have come to this conclusion is uniquely my own experience. It may not happen to you—I have heard from clients and friends alike about how much they miss their bustling lives before long Covid, how they mourn the life experience that they have now lost as a cause of their illness. I still can empathize—I know what that loss feels like, even if I do not mourn it.

Instead, I have preferred to stay in the moment, rather than race onto the next one. I'm much more deliberate in my actions. I've lowered my bar on certain expectations, which has not been such a bad thing.

In a related sense, long Covid motivated me to downsize my life. I have lost the taste I had for material goods, for the material world. I still like material goods, of course, but I am just not as quick to buy into the lifestyle that requires material commodities. My Covid recovery experiment has led me to a modest life right now, and I will see where the coming years take me.

Now, peace of mind has become a commodity. Mindfulness has become a commodity. Compassion has become a commodity. Forgiveness has become a commodity. Gratitude has become a commodity. There are extraordinary research studies on practicing daily gratitude as a means of building better brain capacity. I used to ignore the reparative benefits of gratitude mediation, foolishly.

So have I changed? Yes. I was the son of very poor Cuban immigrants, I received my education in the New York City public schools, and I grew up full of ambition, eager to accumulate wealth, power, and prestige.

Through my journey, I have become a different version of me—perhaps a more authentic version and a more thoughtful, mindful, and grateful one. I've seen a transformation of my character, and sometimes it can be hard to fathom.

You have read through my experiences, you know what it took for me to recover, and I want you to learn from me. I may not be immortal but I have survived and feel quite well most days. It's hard work to stay healthy, yet now's a good time to reexamine your lifestyle and recognize that discipline is perhaps the most unlikely of allies.

I believe now, in light of much of the current science and daily revelations, that much of my plan offers guidelines for living a good life, beyond just accelerating past long Covid syndrome and the challenges it may bring.

I thought I was immortal, but nobody is. I hope my story and the recommendations I have made will help you in your journey and prepare you for the coming variants. I believe we are living in a challenging moment in the history of the world and anything you can do to reinforce your immune system, train your mind, develop discipline, and strengthen your spirit will prepare you for whatever may come your way.

Remember, always, that we are all in this together.

—Oz Garcia

LONG COVID SYMPTOM LIST

Long Covid still remains an enigmatic force throughout the world of medicine. It is a chronic illness with symptoms ranging from cognitive problems, fatigue, gastrointestinal issues, unexpected responses to exercise, and much more. While there have been spectacular advances in the field of vaccination and infection prevention, the research surrounding the long term effects of Covid have largely been open ended. The reason for this lies in the unknown magnitude of the virus. There is no historical comparison for a respiratory virus this potent and transmissible. Long Covid has become a problem whose power comes from its variance and opaqueness. However, there have been ample studies done to show some of the most common symptoms of long Covid.

Long Covid has been confirmed as a medical condition by the CDC's Dr. Anthony Fauci and the medical community at large. In general, Covid becomes long Covid once one's symptoms extend beyond the standard incubation period. The evidence suggests that long Covid does not discriminate based on the original virus variant contracted. There have been documented cases of long

Covid from Beta, Delta, and Omicron alike. Although certain viral infections, like influenza, have been well documented to, at times, contain post-viral ailments, the symptoms of long Covid are decidedly more drastic, and often harder to explain. Long Covid symptoms can also often go unseen in a conventional medical testing setting. It is abundantly clear that long Covid sufferers and their struggles have not been heard, as evidenced by the CDC's small list of long Covid symptoms compared to the list that has been procured by various studies. Here is the list of long Covid symptoms that we know of:

Symptoms of long Covid

FATIGUE
- Severe fatigue
- Struggle with physical activity
- Myalgic encephalomyelitis/Chronic Fatigue Syndrome (ME/CFS)

IMMUNE
- Disrupted immune system function
- Lasting, damaging autoimmune response
- General inflammation

CIRCULATORY
- Circulatory system dysfunction
- Impaired oxygen flow
- Vascular damage and blood clots
- Muscle aches

- Dysautonomia
- Heart palpitations
- Tachycardia (irregular heartbeat)
- Loss of stamina while exercising

BRAIN

- Brain fog
- Nerve fiber damage (small fiber neuropathy)
- Brain inflammation and low oxygen levels
- Oxygen flow limitation
- Cognitive impairment
- Reduced attention, memory, communicative efficacy
- Reduced blood flow to the brain
- Difficulty concentrating
- Memory recall speed and efficiency
- General confusion

MENTAL BARRIERS

- Anxiety
- Depression or prolonged periods of sadness
- Irritability

LUNGS

- Shortness of breath
- Lung damage
- Decreased lung function

DIGESTIVE TRACT

- Indigestion/bowel discomfort
- Acid reflux/heartburn

SLEEP

- Sleep disturbance
- Night sweats
- Oversleeping

SIGHT/SMELL/HEARING/TASTE

- Blurry vision
- Floaters
- Dry eyes
- Partial or complete loss of sense of smell
- Clogged ears
- Tinnitus
- Partial or complete loss of taste

NERVOUS SYSTEM

- Tremors
- Muscle twitching

PAIN

- Persistent chest pain
- Joint pain
- Muscle and body aches
- Abdominal pain
- Lower back pain
- Upper back pain
- Sharp and sudden chest pain

COLD SYMPTOMS

- Cough
- Sore throat
- Fever or chills

- Congestion
- Calf cramping

OTHER

- Nausea or vomiting
- Weight gain
- Skin rashes
- Headache
- Dizziness
- Hair loss

ACKNOWLEDGMENTS

The gratitude I feel for the many people who helped in the creation of this book begins with my parents. As Cuban immigrants, the resilience they demonstrated in their lives was instilled in me and gave me the essential grit to survive. My mother, in particular, always rose above her circumstances. In my darkest moments, I turn to the memory of her which strengthens my resolve. My brother Albert, too, has always had my back. No one matches him in the deeply-appreciated support he's given me all these years. The amazing Paulina, whose love has never wavered, thank you. I couldn't have made it this far without the consistent inspiration exhibited by: Freddy, and his belief in me and this project; Tara, who makes sure I'm always where I should be; Danielle, my foil, supreme project manager and relentless champion of all our causes; the infinitely reliable Samir, king of our clinic and dispenser of magical cures; Leila and her wonderful husband, Alberto, whom we lost too soon and too early in the war against Covid; my publisher Judith Regan, who, from day one, saw my vision and has supported me through the trials I underwent to get this project launched and into the world; Betsy Perry who got me started putting my story together; the incomparable and dedicated Henry Schwartz who dove in with such commitment and skill and helped me write the book in record time—so many thanks to you; Stephen Meringoff, without his true and undeniable support, I wouldn't be here—his unfailing support saved me as Covid took hold and ravaged my body and helped so much in pulling me back to life. And thank you, with all of my heart, to the countless and nameless doctors, nurses, and health care workers of all kinds who showered me with love, support, and optimism in my darkest moments.

ABOUT THE AUTHORS

OZ GARCIA is recognized as an authority on healthy aging, age reversal, and fortifying the immune system in the age of Covid. His client list includes A-List celebrities, Fortune 500 CEOs, and, more recently, those dealing with Covid and post-Covid health issues. Oz Garcia's unique and customized approach to nutrition, functional health, and self-optimization, combined with more than forty years of experience, has made him one of the most recognizable names in the industry. Garcia has lectured worldwide and is known as a trailblazer in the study of nutrition, ensuring quality of life as we age, and learning to survive Covid by creating a strong immune system.

Oz is the bestselling author of four books: *The Food Cure for Kids*, *The Balance*, *Look and Feel Fabulous Forever*, and *Redesigning 50: The No-Plastic-Surgery Guide to 21st-Century Age Defiance*. He was twice voted best nutritionist by *New York* magazine and is frequently called upon by some of the most respected names in medicine and media for his up-to-the-minute views on nutrition and its role in aging and longevity. Oz has been featured in *Vogue, Elle, Travel and Leisure, W* magazine, and the *New York Times*. He has also made numerous television appearances, including on NBC's *The Today Show,* CBS's *This Morning,* ABC's *Good Morning America, 20/20, 48 Hours,* Fox News, and *The View*.

HENRY SCHWARTZ is a writer from Los Angeles.

9 781682 452035